# A Patient's Guide to
# ACOUSTIC NEUROMA

# A Patient's Guide to
# ACOUSTIC NEUROMA

Mark Knoblauch PhD

Kiremma Press
Houston, TX

Disclaimer: The information provided within this book is for general informational purposes only. While we try to keep the information up-to-date and correct, there are no representations or warranties, express or implied, about the completeness, accuracy, reliability, suitability or availability with respect to the information contained in this book for any purpose. Any use of this information is at your own risk. Furthermore, the methods described within this book are the author's personal thoughts and opinions. As such, they are not intended to be a definitive set of instructions for you to follow precisely. You may discover there are other methods and materials to accomplish the same end result.

www.authorMK.com

ISBN: 978-1-7320674-8-6

*For all those who have had to deal with the fear and uncertainty associated with any vestibular condition*

# Table of Contents

# Introduction

Living with any condition that results in dizziness, hearing loss, unsteadiness, or vertigo can have a significant impact on an individual's life. Even more frustrating is that a patient's initial suspicions as to the source of these symptoms can include terrifying possibilities such as stroke or seizure. Only after what can often be many physician visits does a patient receive word that the source of their symptoms is not a brain disorder but rather a condition localized to their inner-ear. While learning that a disease exists can be troublesome, once armed with a final diagnosis, patients can begin a focused and dedicated treatment plan that can reduce or eliminate their symptoms and improve their overall condition.

Inner ear disorders come in many shapes and sizes. Some conditions such as the presence of tinnitus are apt to cause a degree of frustration, while others such as Ménière's disease or vestibular migraine can cause a complete disruption to one's way of life. Unfortunately, many of these vestibular disorders occur without a clear understanding of their cause. And without a clearly identified cause, treatments are unable to focus on the true source of the problem and are instead geared more toward controlling the associated symptoms.

Acoustic neuroma differs from many other inner ear disorders in that they are a physical, benign tumor that can be clearly identified through techniques such as magnetic resonance imaging (MRI). The fact that acoustic neuromas are a physical mass probably plays a role in the long history that acoustic neuroma has been afforded in medicine, a stark contrast to some of the other inner ear conditions such as vestibular migraine or benign paroxysmal positional vertigo (BPPV) which have only gained attention over the past 20 years or so. As such, much of the information we have on acoustic neuroma has been known for the past 70 years or more, with new information helping to sharpen our existing understanding of the condition.

As a patient of many inner-ear disorders myself, I have found a passion of sorts in providing patients a reliable and understandable reference guide specific to their vestibular diagnosis. Having lived with Ménière's disease, BPPV, and tinnitus, I am familiar with days consumed by dizziness and vertigo, and how those symptoms can have a tremendous impact on your daily life. What was particularly frustrating for me during my various diagnoses was that I could not find what I felt was a quality, factual overview of the condition I was dealing with. I found several sources that pushed me toward miracle cures or paid websites, but that wasn't in any way the type of information I was in the mood for at the time. Rather, I was seeking information that outlined what my condition was, how it came to be, and most importantly – how to fix it. In short, I wanted to be educated on my condition, with information based on research and facts rather than personal opinion and anecdotes. And that drive has led me to write several books on vestibular conditions, with this acoustic neuroma book being my latest project.

I feel quite confident that the vast majority of acoustic neuroma patients – particularly those who are newly diagnosed – are seeking a similar level of information when dealing with a disease as unfamiliar to them as acoustic neuroma. They are most likely looking for quality information specific to medical procedures, diagnosis, treatment, and quality of life. After all, it's not like acoustic neuroma patients have found out that they have some common condition such as a broken bone or an infection; rather, they are dealing with the fact that a tumor exists within their inner ear – something that they are probably both quite unfamiliar and uncomfortable with. If you as an acoustic neuroma patient are anything like me, the uncertainty of an unknown but significant disease leads you to want to find out as much information as you can about the condition.

That inherent desire for information is what this book is all about. It is written to serve as a comprehensive patient guide that details several aspects of your interaction with acoustic neuroma. We will begin with an overview of the relevant inner ear and brain anatomy associated with acoustic neuroma so as to highlight the main structures involved. Next, we will focus on the condition of acoustic neuroma itself, looking at relevant terminology, its incidence and prevalence, suspected causes, and the relevant symptoms. Then, we will spend a chapter outlining the diagnostic procedures used, in order to detail out for you the testing procedures commonly used in identification of acoustic neuroma. We will follow that up with a chapter describing the various treatments associated with acoustic neuroma, discussing the various recommendations specific to conservative and more invasive treatments, even detailing out several treatment procedures. We'll then look at quality of life aspects for acoustic neuroma patients, focusing on the expected outcomes for the many treatment options available. Finally, our closing chapter serves to outline several medical conditions that exhibit signs and symptoms similar to acoustic neuroma in order to help you recognize the similarities as well as differences of each.

This book is designed to provide you vital information that you need as a patient of acoustic neuroma. What you will find is the latest research, backed up with citations of pertinent facts so that you yourself can investigate further any particular areas of interest. What you won't find are personal opinions from me as the author, or sales pitches for some product I'm hyping. My goal is to provide you a quality source of information to better inform you about your condition.

What you do with that information is up to you. It may be that you have a more informed dialogue with your medical professional. Or perhaps you give this book to a friend or family member who doesn't understand or feel empathetic to your situation. Regardless of what you do with the information provided in this book, it is my intent as the author of this patient guide to leave you better informed and more assertive as a patient of acoustic neuroma so that you can pursue the best treatment and ensure the most productive quality of life available.

Now, let's begin your journey to learning more about acoustic neuroma.

# Chapter 1: Anatomy of the ear

While it might be of interest to dive right into the intricacies of acoustic neuroma, I think it better that we first outline the underlying anatomy and physiology involved with this condition. In doing so, it can help provide you a relevant background that can serve as a foundation for the next chapter that specifically targets what an acoustic neuroma is as well as how it affects us. By reviewing the anatomy associated with acoustic neuroma you will be able to visualize the affected structures and be able to differentiate many of the associated components of the middle ear. So while this chapter may seem somewhat like an anatomy book at times, its real purpose is to provide you a solid foundation behind not only the anatomy involved in acoustic neuroma but also those structures that provide information to the brain specific to our movements and body position.

The rationale for being all-inclusive with the anatomy of the ear is that when these balance-related structures are functioning incorrectly, we are left with what ends up being some of the symptoms of acoustic neuroma – vertigo, imbalance, and dizziness. Therefore, this chapter will highlight not only the major components of our inner ear but also outline how several of these structures are responsible for our ability to maintain balance and equilibrium.

## Sections of the ear

*Outer ear*

The most noticeable aspect of what we commonly characterize as our 'ear' is the portion that we can see (Figure 1.1). This includes the large pinna as well as the ear canal that leads to the eardrum, which collectively makes up our outer ear. The function of the outer ear is largely limited to funneling sound into the eardrum, and as it is located well away from the inner ear structures that are involved with acoustic neuroma, the outer ear is not considered to have any involvement with the development or outcomes of acoustic neuroma.

*Middle ear*

The middle ear is the air-filled portion of the ear located behind the eardrum and housed within the temporal bone (Figure 1.1). This portion of the ear holds the three small bones – the malleus, stapes, and incus – that transfer sound from the eardrum to the inner ear. The most association you will likely have with the middle ear is when you suffer the effects of an ear infection. As the middle ear is really nothing more than a space within the temporal bone, it has no specific involvement with acoustic neuroma.

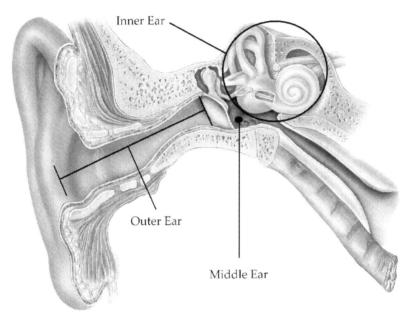

Inner Ear

Outer Ear

Middle Ear

*Figure 1.1. The three sections of the ear include the outer ear, middle ear, and inner ear. Issues involved with acoustic neuroma influence signals that are sent from this labyrinth portion of the inner ear*

## Inner ear

The inner ear is responsible for two major roles in our body. First, it detects and converts sound waves to neural impulses. In other words, it is responsible for our sense of hearing. While this is certainly no small feat, the inner ear also plays a role in the perception and interpretation of body positioning. This in turn makes the inner ear the site of both our main balance organ as well as our hearing organ.

Because of the intricate roles it has specific to hearing and motion detection, the inner ear is comprised of an array of highly sensitive structures. The sensitivity of these structures also makes the inner ear quite susceptible to injury. Despite its small size, intricate structure, and dual responsibility for handling detection of both sound and motion, damage to the sensitive components of the inner ear can affect hearing as well as equilibrium. Furthermore, even minor disruptive events can trigger several symptoms such as motion sickness, vertigo or nausea. Because of the high level of involvement of the inner ear structures in detecting sound and motion, the inner ear has been called one of the most intensively studied areas of vertebrate anatomy and physiology[1].

There are two main areas that make up the inner ear – the cochlea and the vestibular system. Together, these two structures make up what is known as the *labyrinth*. Despite what you often see in images of the inner ear, the labyrinth organs are not free-standing organs; rather, they are simply tunnels that exist deep within the temporal bone (Figure 1.2). These tunnels contain membranes that serve to contain the unique fluid (i.e. 'endolymph') housed within the labyrinth. As we will discuss, it is the movement of this fluid within the vestibular system that provides much of our ability to detect certain motions of the head.

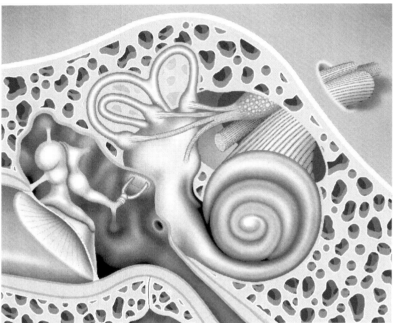

*Figure 1.2  The labyrinth system does not consist of free-standing structures but rather a group of hollowed-out areas of the temporal bone that form a series of cavities and tunnels*

## The vestibular system

Although the inner ear isn't specifically implicated in acoustic neuroma, many of its components play a role in the associated symptoms of acoustic neuroma such as hearing loss and dizziness. Furthermore, the organs of the inner ear send their signals (e.g. hearing, balance) along the vestibular nerve which is known to be the source of an acoustic neuroma. Therefore, we will take a detailed look at the structure and function of these vestibular components thought to play a role in the symptoms associated with acoustic neuroma.

There are two primary systems at play within the inner ear (Figure 1.3). The first is the cochlea, a snail-shaped organ designed to convert sound waves to electrical signals that can be interpreted by the brain as 'sound'. While there is some aspect of hearing loss involved in acoustic neuroma, there is relatively little direct involvement with the cochlea other than an expectation for diminished hearing over time. As such, in this chapter we'll focus predominantly on the vestibular system given its strong link to the symptoms that commonly occur in response to vestibular neuroma.

In terms of an overall purpose, the vestibular system of the inner ear has a primary role of detecting motion of the head, along with serving to provide feedback specific to an individual's head position. It is known that some structures of the vestibular system are involved in acoustic neuroma, and as a result, patients often experience vestibular-related consequences when the acoustic neuroma reaches a particular size. Therefore, I feel it's best that we take a comprehensive look at the components of the vestibular system in order to help you understand how aspects such as unsteadiness or vertigo – both commonly associated with acoustic neuroma –

may develop. To do this, we first need to outline the anatomy of our vestibular system as well as the physiology of how these structures work to provide feedback specific to our head's movement and position.

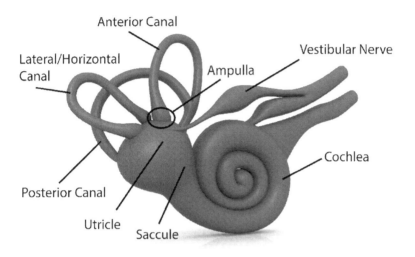

*Figure 1.3. The labyrinth system is comprised of several individual organs including the cochlea, vestibule, and semicircular canals.*

Vestibular anatomy

Five independent structures are involved in our ability to detect motion. The first two structures are housed within an organ termed the vestibule, a 3-5mm wide structure located between the cochlea and semicircular canals. The vestibule itself contains two very important components called the *saccule* and the *utricle* that are responsible for detecting motion that occurs in a linear direction (i.e. forward/backward, up/down, side-to-side). Activities such as running, walking, standing up, or even riding in an elevator are detected by the saccule and the utricle, both of which have thousands of small crystals embedded within their structure to help detect inertia, which is then processed by the brain as movement of the head. Because the saccule and utricle house these small crystals known as *otoliths*, the utricle and saccule are known as the "otolith organs".

In addition to the saccule and utricle, the remainder of the vestibular portion of the inner ear is comprised of three canals called semicircular canals that form loops through the temporal bone. These canals detect circular motion, the kind generated when you shake your head 'yes' or 'no'. The semicircular canals also play a very important role in ensuring that our eyes can stay on a fixed spot or target even while our head is moving.

Without all of these structures functioning properly, our ability to maintain balance and have a normal equilibrium would be severely impaired. As we will outline, many of the symptoms of acoustic neuroma result from an improperly functioning vestibular system in that either the system itself is not working or – more likely – the signals sent from the vestibular system to the brain are impaired due to the presence of the neuroma. To help clarify how all of these components interact, we will take a look at the structures of the vestibular system as well as outline how they work in helping us to detect movement and maintain equilibrium.

## Saccule

The saccule is a bulged-out portion of the vestibule responsible for detecting vertical motion of the head (and with movement of the head typically comes movement of the body as well). For example, jumping up and down or riding in an elevator are activities that stimulate the motion sensors within the saccule. Inside the saccule is a structure called the *macula sacculi*, a vertically-oriented organ which houses a two- to three-millimeter area comprised of sensory hair cells responsible for detecting head motion. The ends of these hair cells extend horizontally into the middle of the vestibule and are covered by a gelatinous layer, over which is a fibrous structure called the otolithic membrane. This otolithic membrane is embedded with thousands of calcium-based crystals known by a variety of names including *statoconia, otoconia,* and the aforementioned *otolith*. For the purpose of this book we will use the term *otolith* to describe the crystals of the ear.

Because it is embedded with otoliths, the otolithic membrane is heavier than the material surrounding it. Therefore, when the body moves somewhat quickly in a vertical plane such as occurs when jumping, gravity pulls the otoliths downward the same way as a leafy branch might bend when you swing it upward. The weight of the otoliths causes nerve cells that extend into the otolithic membrane to bend in response to the linear motion. This in turn causes those hair cells to send a signal to the brain that is interpreted as vertical movement of the head.

## Utricle

The utricle has an almost identical makeup as the saccule but has a slightly different orientation and function. The utricle is larger than the saccule and serves to detect when the head moves in the horizontal plane. Such movements, which occur with forward, backward, or side-to-side motion of the head, happen with walking, running, or even riding in a car. Like the saccule, the utricle contains a macula called the *macula utriculi*. In contrast to the saccule's vertically-oriented macula, the macula utriculi is positioned horizontally with hair cells that are oriented vertically. The mechanism by which the macula utriculi detects motion operates similarly to that of the macula sacculi in that the hair cells are covered with a gelatinous layer which is in turn overlaid with a gel-like membrane embedded with otoliths.

Similar to the vertical action within the saccule, when forward, backward, or side-to-side head motion occurs within the utricle, the inertia created from the force of the motion upon the embedded otoliths creates a sort of 'shearing' motion between the gelatinous layer and the otolithic membrane. This motion is then detected by the utricle's embedded nerve cells which in turn send a signal to the brain that gets interpreted as a specific horizontal movement of the head.

## Semicircular Canals

In addition to the vestibule's saccule and utricle structures, there are three semicircular canals of the inner ear's labyrinth network that make up the remainder of the vestibular system. As mentioned earlier, the semicircular canals are not true bony structures themselves; rather, they exist as 'tunnels' or canals through the temporal bone. Thin membranes line the bone-encased semicircular canals and serve to contain fluid known as endolymph that is found throughout the labyrinth system. Like each maculi of the utricle and saccule that detect linear movement, rotational or 'angular' motions of the head cause this endolymph to move within the canals – a process that we will discuss shortly. An example of angular motion would include turning the head side-to-side as if watching a tennis match. Because this movement does not generate enough inertia within the inner ear to act upon the saccule or utricle, the design of the semicircular canals allow them to detect this angular motion as the endolymph flows across specialized sensors within each canal. The brain then interprets the signal from these sensors to establish the direction of head movement.

There are three independent semicircular canals – the anterior, posterior, and horizontal canals. The placement of the three canals positions them at right angles to each other which in turn allows all head motions to be detected. This design can be imagined by thinking of a corner of a cube – each of the three sides of the cube represents a different plane of movement similar to how any angular movement of the head can be detected by one or more of the semicircular canals.

So how does movement of fluid within the semicircular canals actually result in the brain being able to detect the motion? It's quite a fascinating process (at least in my mind!), actually. Angular motion is detected due to endolymph passing over a specialized organ within each canal called the *cupula*. Movement of the head in an angular motion (i.e. shaking the head 'no', nodding the head, etc.) causes movement of endolymph, which in turn flows across hair cells that move in response to the flow of endolymph. These hair cells are located within the canal itself, at each end of the semicircular canal in a bulged-out area called the *ampulla* (see Figure 1.3). Hair cells within the ampulla contain the cupula, a gelatinous layer over the hair cells that extends across the width of the ampulla.

Let's look at this process in a little more detail. When a person moves his or her head, the endolymph moves within the semicircular canal in response to the head movement. As the fluid moves, it flows around the cupula (Figure 1.4). As the fluid motion of the endolymph pushes against the cupula, the cupula bends in response to the fluid moving over it. This causes hair cells immediately under the cupula to also bend, the same way we described that tree branch bending if its leafy end were placed into flowing water. This bending of the hair cells sends a signal to the brain which is interpreted as motion appropriate to the direction of head movement.

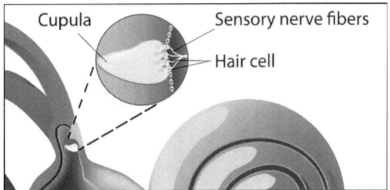

*Figure 1.4. Near the end of each semicircular canal, the ampulla houses the sensitive cupula organ which is responsible for detecting movement of fluid within the respective semicircular canal*

These events occurring within the semicircular canals are important to understand, as they are largely thought to play a role in vertigo and dizziness. As far back as the 1960s, researchers believed that conditions such as benign paroxysmal positional vertigo (BPPV) – which triggers bouts of vertigo, nystagmus (rapid eye motion), and unsteadiness – resulted from otoliths pressing against the cupula within the semicircular canal[2]. This interference was suspected of increasing the cupula's sensitivity to motion, in turn generating the symptoms associated with BPPV.

## The vestibulocochlear nerve

Now that you know how all of the various balance detectors work, you can better understand the complications that may arise when the vestibular nerve gets compressed by an acoustic neuroma. As the acoustic neuroma grows, it begins to press against the vestibular nerve. This in turn inhibits the nerve's ability to send signals from the various movement sensors (i.e. semicircular canals, vestibule) of the inner ear, causing the brain to get inadequate or mixed signals that can then lead to physical manifestations including imbalance, dizziness, and even vertigo. Again, even though the sensors are working properly within the vestibular system, the ability to transmit messages about head position from those sensors to the brain is compromised. This in turn results in many of the symptoms associated with acoustic neuroma such as imbalance and dizziness. And compression of the vestibulocochlear nerve may contribute in part to other symptoms of acoustic neuroma such as tinnitus and hearing loss (Figure 1.5). Because of the vestibular nerve's involvement in acoustic neuroma we'll now focus our attention on the vestibular nerve itself in order to outline the nerve's location and function, which will in turn help us understand how it is affected when an acoustic neuroma occurs.

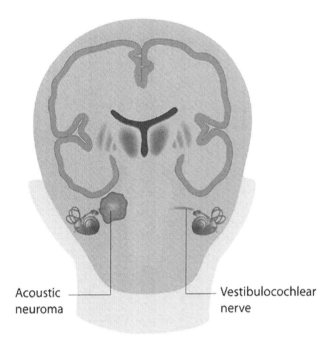

Acoustic neuroma

Vestibulocochlear nerve

*Figure 1.5. The vestibulocochlear nerve is responsible for sending signals from the hearing and balance detectors of each inner ear over to the brain, and is the tissue source of an acoustic neuroma*

The vestibulocochlear nerve has been previously known by other names that include *auditory nerve* and *acoustic nerve*. These names, however, fail to represent the main function of the nerve, which is to relay signals from the vestibular system to the brain. As such, the term *vestibulocochlear nerve* is most commonly used these days. The nerve itself is one of the 12 cranial nerves designed to provide movement and sensation to various areas of the head and upper body. As a cranial nerve, the vestibulocochlear nerve is characterized by Roman

31

numeral VIII, or "8", leading to it often being described as "cranial nerve VIII". Although it is largely considered as one nerve, it originates as two independent sections within the labyrinth portion of the inner ear – the aforementioned vestibular system as well as the cochlear nerve that transmits messages from the hearing-focused cochlea to the brain.

*The Schwann cell*

Many nerve cells within the body produce a specialized cell type called *myelin*. In nerve cells, myelin is produced to form a 'sheath' around the outside of the nerve fiber that serves to not only insulate the nerve but also help to increase the speed at which a nerve signal is transmitted. Therefore, myelinated nerves can transmit their signals faster than unmyelinated nerves. The cell type that produces myelin is known as a Schwann cell. Interestingly, acoustic neuromas are more commonly known as *acoustic schwannoma* or *vestibular schwannoma* given that this terminology better emphasizes its origination from Schwann cells of the vestibular nerve (and '-oma' is usually tacked on to the end to indicate tumor growth). During the early growth phase of a nerve, a point is reached at which it makes a transition from generating nerve tissue to producing this outer level of myelinated tissue. It is at this point that Schwann cells are activated. As we will discuss later, something appears to occur within this Schwann cell portion of the nerve to trigger growth of an acoustic neuroma.

## The facial nerve

In a book about acoustic neuroma, it's relevant to talk not only about the vestibulocochlear nerve but also another adjacent cranial nerve known as the facial nerve (i.e. cranial nerve VII, or "7"). As we will outline in later chapters, the facial nerve is susceptible to compression (and subsequent diminished function) from an acoustic neuroma and is also at risk for injury from acoustic neuroma surgery.

The facial nerve's pathway from the base of the brain takes it alongside the vestibulocochlear nerve through an opening in the skull called the *internal acoustic meatus*. As it reaches the exterior and frontal portion of the skull (i.e. the 'face'), the facial nerve branches out into several sections that help provide movement to the muscles of the face (Figure 1.6). Therefore, the facial nerve has a vital role in providing our ability to create facial expressions (which explains its prior name as the *expressive* nerve)[3]. But its responsibility does not end there, as it also controls a muscle within our middle ear that helps regulate the activity of the stirrup bone, in turn preventing unnecessary vibration within our cochlea that can be caused by loud noise[3]. Similarly, the facial nerve is responsible for detecting sensation around our outer ear as well as around the eardrum. The facial nerve also generates the reflex that causes us to blink when any object touches our cornea[3]. And the facial nerve even plays a role in taste perception, as one segment of the nerve is responsible for relaying taste from the front two-thirds of our tongue[3]. Clearly, the facial nerve has a major role in our daily life.

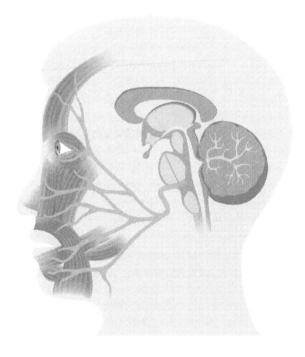

*Figure 1.6. The facial nerve has several roles including the regulation of multiple muscles located around the facial area*

The fact that our facial nerve has so much responsibility is probably why acoustic neuroma patients are quite intent on ensuring that their facial nerve function is retained, especially given the fact that certain acoustic neuroma treatments such as surgery can increase the risk for damage to the nerve. Think about it, how might a loss of your ability to make facial expressions – or at least the ability to make expressions on the affected side of your face – impact your self-confidence or your quality of life. At what point would the symptoms of acoustic neuroma be worth the risk of losing this ability, or the ability to taste and/or feel sensation in the facial area? This is a risk that many acoustic neuroma patients must face, and given the important role of the facial nerve, it is a decision that should involve a deep discussion with the patient and their physician.

## Vertigo and the vestibular system

The preceding portion of this chapter has outlined in detail much about the vestibular system as well as relevant cranial nerves that we rely on for daily function. My reasoning for going into such detail with each is two-fold. First, I want you to have an understanding of the complexity of the vestibular system, for as we have discussed, this system is quite intricate. Even a small disruption to the vestibular system can have a significant impact on several aspects of our life. The extent of this impact leads to the second reason I wanted to outline the vestibular system in depth – to help you understand the mechanisms involved in balance and vertigo that can arise as a result of acoustic neuroma.

As mentioned earlier, the vestibulocochlear nerve is not only the location of acoustic neuroma, it is also responsible for transmitting signals from the vestibular system to the brain. Even in cases where the movement and balance detectors (i.e. semicircular canals, saccule, utricle) are functioning normally, adequate processing of the signals that these structures send is dependent upon that signal reaching the brain. With acoustic neuroma, we will be discussing in the next chapter how growth of the neuroma can put pressure against the vestibulocochlear nerve, which in turn can limit the amount of signal being sent through the nerve to the brain. This of course can lead to symptoms such as imbalance and/or dizziness due to the brain not being able to properly interpret the signal. And while imbalance or unsteadiness is problematic enough, up to half of acoustic neuroma patients report experiencing vertigo attacks[4]. Therefore, to help patients understand the link between acoustic neuroma and vertigo we will next discuss the event of vertigo itself.

Vertigo is the sensation of movement when in fact no movement is occurring. It is important to understand that vertigo is a symptom – not an actual medical condition; therefore, expecting a cure for vertigo is effectively the same as expecting a cure for pain. What is likely meant is that one expects a cure for what is *causing* the vertigo. Vertigo itself is largely thought to result from events occurring within the inner ear, and other medical conditions that trigger vertigo – such as BPPV – are known to originate from within the inner ear. Still, other vertigo-inducing conditions are not as clear cut and are thought to involve a complex interaction between the brain (i.e. 'central' type vertigo) and the inner ear (i.e. 'peripheral' vertigo).

As a patient of a vestibular-related condition it is important to understand that vertigo has several possible sources, and no one event or structure has been established as a primary cause for vertigo. However, researchers have largely narrowed peripheral vertigo down to the semicircular canals, saccule, or utricle, while central vertigo is typically associated with either the brainstem or the vestibulocochlear nerve[5]. When functioning normally, the inner ear structures send signals to the brain in a coordinated pattern from the left and right ear. However, an imbalance of these vestibular inputs – such as can occur when one of our two vestibular systems is not performing correctly – leads to uncoordinated information being transmitted to the brain, in turn triggering events such as nystagmus (rapid and uncontrollable eye movement) or vertigo to occur. This imbalanced signal can occur due to disruption anywhere along the neural pathway that stretches from the vestibular-based sensors to the brain.

Again, there is no specific structure or area that triggers vertigo across all patients. Therefore, vertigo can arise from multiple causes and conditions. For example, patients experiencing migraine (i.e. a specific type of headache) sometimes experience vertigo similar to patients with a disorder specific to the vestibule of the inner ear. Sometimes vertigo even originates outside of the skull, such as can occur in patients who experience vertigo that results from degrading intervertebral discs, a condition known as 'cervical vertigo'[6].

One confounding issue that medical professionals have in establishing vertigo is that patients often lump it in with dizziness. Both vertigo and dizziness are indeed similar in their effects given that each can make you as the patient feel unsteady. One recommended way to separate the two conditions is to outline whether you feel 'lightheaded' or whether you feel as though the world is spinning around you. Generally, a spinning sensation is more characteristic of vertigo, while lightheadedness is typically associated with dizziness[7].

Vertigo occurs when the patient reports that their world is spinning around them despite the fact that they are stationary. So what exactly causes this sensation? Physiologically speaking, the sensation of vertigo is largely due to a link between the inner ear and the eyes. While this may seem to be a somewhat odd link, the interconnection between our ears and eyes plays a vital role in our daily function even though we may not recognize it (until there is a problem!). To outline this role, we need to discuss the vestibulo-ocular reflex (VOR) and how it coordinates the interaction between the ear and eye.

# The vestibulo-ocular reflex (VOR)

Although our eyes have independent functions specific to providing our sense of vision, they are intimately connected with the inner ear. This interaction plays an important role in our ability to maintain balance as well as to maintain acuity when we are moving. To see how important your vision is for aiding in your balance, walk quickly from a bright room into a very dark one. You'll probably find that you are initially timid and a little bit unsteady, which will likely improve once your eyes adjust to the darkness. Similarly, jump up and down a few times and notice how your vision of the field around you is still quite clear and steady – a stark contrast from watching a video that was recorded on camera you held while jumping. The ability to maintain this smooth field of vision even while engaged in strenuous activity such as jumping is because of the intricate link between the vestibular system and movement of the eyes. In fact, this link has even been given a name – the 'vestibulo-ocular reflex' (VOR). We won't go deep into the details of how the VOR works, but we will next provide a general overview of the reflex as it relates to a few expected symptoms of acoustic neuroma.

The interconnection between your vestibular system and eyes is what allows you to maintain a smooth, non-jumpy field of vision while running or riding on a bumpy road. This happens because the vestibular system actually has some control over the muscle of the eyes through the VOR that allows your eyes to remain fixed on an object even though your head position may be moving. This reflex has the task of trying to ensure that an image or object remains stable on an individual's retina in order to allow for proper processing by the brain[8]. Without the VOR, every time your head moves, you would consciously need to readjust your eye position back to the object you are looking at. With the VOR, however, your vestibular system is able to detect the speed of your head motion and automatically control the muscles in your eye so that your gaze easily remains fixed on the object. This reflex also works well when driving, as every time you hit a bump or turn a corner your eyes are subconsciously controlled by the VOR rather than jumping all around while trying to manually reposition – which would certainly be a problem when operating a vehicle!

When the VOR is working correctly you don't even know that it's there. But when there is a disruption to the system – such as occurs in response to a vestibular-related disease such as acoustic neuroma – the VOR becomes impaired and can lead to uncontrolled movements such as the aforementioned nystagmus. Consequently, an affected patient is not able to coordinate their eye movements with the movements of their head. This can lead to jumpy or blurry vision, likely occurring most often when the head is moving or the patient's body is in motion. Another condition that can result is *oscillopia*, a condition in which objects in the field of vision appear to float around even though they are in fact stationary, due in large part to the muscles of the eye being unable to keep the eye adequately fixed on one object.

Additional problems occur when a person with a faulty VOR tries to follow movement or read text on paper or a computer screen, an event known as *tracking*. With the VOR not allowing for smooth eye movement such as that required to follow a thrown ball or read printed text, it can be difficult for the patient to make the smooth eye motions needed to properly intake visual information (i.e. identify and process the written words). Without a well-established link between our eyes and our ears, life would be much more difficult. But unfortunately, because of this link between our eyes and ears we must often pay the price of having visual disturbances such as vertigo or nystagmus when our vestibular system is malfunctioning.

## Conclusion

Clearly, the inner ear consists of highly intricate and complex structures. Without a properly functioning vestibular system, our ability to maintain posture, recognize our movements, and sense positional changes can be extremely difficult. The intent of this chapter was to provide an overview of those structural components of the inner ear involved in acoustic neuroma. In addition, we touched on several physiological processes that can occur in response to an acoustic neuroma such as vertigo. Understand that what we covered in this chapter is indeed quite generic in scope; there is in fact much, much more that we could discuss at a much deeper level. However, as I stated early on my focus is to keep this book oriented as a guide for acoustic neuroma patients rather than serving as a medical textbook. What you will hopefully find is that as you continue to read subsequent chapters, the detailed information we have discussed here becomes more relevant to you given that you better understand the various anatomy and physiology of the inner ear. Now, we'll spend the remainder of this book outlining various aspects of acoustic neuroma, starting with the next chapter where we'll characterize the main aspects of the condition itself – who it affects, its suspected causes, and the most common symptoms.

# Chapter 2 – Acoustic Neuroma

Understanding the anatomy of the inner ear provides us a framework for recognizing those main structures that are involved with acoustic neuroma. With this knowledge we can now shift our focus towards outlining the main premise of this book – what an acoustic neuroma is and how it can affect the patient. In this chapter we'll first take a broad look at acoustic neuroma, including the various terminology used, a brief history of how our understanding of acoustic neuroma has evolved, and who is affected by acoustic neuroma specific to aspects such as gender, age, ethnicity, etc. We'll then dive into the main focus of this chapter by outlining the anatomical and physiological aspects of acoustic neuroma – what it is, its origins and growth, and the factors behind the symptoms that acoustic neuromas can cause. In tackling these topics, it is hoped that this chapter can provide you a basic but inclusive overview of acoustic neuroma specific to what this disease involves, who it affects, and how it affects them. This information will in turn set the groundwork for subsequent chapters that outline the diagnosis and treatment of acoustic neuroma.

## Nomenclature

The condition of acoustic neuroma has been written about in the medical literature for well over a century. Over this time there have been several different terms used to describe the same condition that we have been referring to as an acoustic neuroma. One of the most popular and most accepted terms in the medical literature is *vestibular schwannoma,* a name that is generally preferred due to the fact that it emphasizes how the condition both affects the vestibular nerve and arises from the Schwann cell portion of the nerve. This name contrasts with the term 'acoustic neuroma', which doesn't quite capture the true nature of the condition, particularly that the 'acoustic' component of the title isn't representative of its true origin from within the vestibular nerve.

Another term you might hear used in place of 'acoustic neuroma' is *acoustic neurinoma.* Stedman's medical dictionary defines a neurinoma as both an obsolete term for 'schwannoma' as well as a term for a tumor of any of the body's Schwann cells - not just those we know as acoustic neuroma[9]. Along these lines, you might also hear the term *neoplasm* associated with acoustic neuroma, which is described as any type of mass that occurs as a result of a tissue's cells dividing more than they should.

Given that we are discussing terminology, we should also take a moment to address one of the most charged terms linked with acoustic neuroma – *tumor*. Unfortunately, the word 'tumor' has a powerfully negative effect given its association with cancer, yet the medical literature does in fact use the term 'tumor' quite often in reference to an acoustic neuroma. It is important to understand, though, that acoustic neuroma is considered a benign and non-cancerous tumor and should not be considered cancerous in nature unless specifically identified as such[10].

All of these terms are effectively the same and used to various degrees across the medical literature and reports discusses acoustic neuroma. Because these terms are interchangeable, and in order to avoid excessive repetition, we will for the purposes of this book stick with the more familiar terms *acoustic neuroma, neuroma,* and *tumor* in our descriptions of the mass of tissue commonly referred to as an acoustic neuroma.

# A brief history of acoustic neuroma treatment

As far back as the early 1890s, surgeons were attempting to remove acoustic neuromas from patients.

The consequence of these highly invasive first surgeries, however, was death[11]. In 1895, the first known acoustic neuroma was removed successfully from a pregnant female who just one day later had a successful delivery[12]. Likely due to an unfamiliarity with both the disease as well as a lack of understanding of surgery techniques back then, surgical intervention for acoustic neuromas back in the late 1800s was not favorable, as over 80% of patients who underwent surgery ended up dying[13]. However, as the century turned, improvements in surgical techniques dropped the death rate of acoustic neuroma surgery down to around 20%.

Until the 1950s, detection of acoustic neuroma was largely inferred from signs such as facial numbness or headaches. Tests were available but were quite limited in scope, such as the caloric test that utilized cool or warm water to stimulate the semicircular canals[12]. Eventually, technological advances in both surgical equipment and imaging devices (e.g. MRI, CT) as well as surgical technique improvements over the years dropped the death rate of acoustic neuroma surgery down to our current rate of effectively zero. In addition, advances in non-surgical procedures such as gamma knife radiation along with our improved understanding of conservative treatment outcomes have allowed for viable and effective alternatives to surgery[13].

# What is an acoustic neuroma

In order to gain an understanding of acoustic neuroma as a medical condition, we have to first outline just what the condition is. Acoustic neuromas are just one of many tissue masses that can arise within the skull, including cysts, aneurysms, facial nerve schwannomas, or meningiomas[14]. In order to be classified as an acoustic neuroma though, the neuroma must originate from the cells of the vestibular nerve. This particular nerve is a common site for tumor development, as approximately 90% of intracranial nerve sheath tumors stem from the 8th cranial nerve[15], the same location from where acoustic neuroma originates.

Anatomically speaking, acoustic neuromas are benign (i.e. non-malignant) gray or yellowish masses that arise from both the superior and inferior portion of the vestibular nerve[16]. They are relatively firm and typically grow as an individual tumor, pressing up against other structures rather than invading and intermixing with the neighboring tissue[17]. The structure of a neuroma is generally solid in nature with a rough, irregular surface[17]. As we will later discuss, the determinant of the neuroma's ultimate size can vary, but as an acoustic neuroma grows within the confined space of the skull, its solid nature will almost certainly begin to compress neighboring structures.

# Prevalence and Incidence

In the study of any disease, it is important to understand just how widespread the disease or condition is, along with outlining how many new cases might be expected to arise each year. For example, if a suspected non-harmful substance leaked from a chemical plant, at first it might seem as though there would be nothing to worry about. However, if a year later it was determined that the new cancer diagnosis rate within one mile of that plant was 312% higher than the prior year, this higher incidence rate would make it imperative to establish a cause for the higher rate. By studying how many people are affected by a disease at a point in time (prevalence) as well as how many new cases arise in a year (incidence), it can help provide valuable information into the potential cause of a particular condition. Because a true cause of acoustic neuroma has not been determined, we must continue to study both its prevalence and incidence rates in order to continue to gather data that may eventually help to reveal important information about the cause of these tumors.

Specific to incidence, one of the first studies that looked at incidence rate occurred in Denmark in the early 1990s where it was determined that approximately 10 acoustic neuromas occur per million people[18]. This study provided valuable information as to the expected occurrence rate of acoustic neuroma, and established a baseline that could be used for later comparisons. It is this baseline that has helped make clear that there appears to be an increasing rate of diagnosis of acoustic neuroma as subsequent and broader studies have reported a higher incidence rate – nearly 20 diagnoses of acoustic neuroma per million people per year[19].

While an increase in the incidence of acoustic neuroma might at first sound alarming, there are potential explanations. One reason may simply be due to discrepancies in how prior data was collected on acoustic neuromas. Or it could be explained by the fact that medicine is constantly developing better technology that allows practitioners to more easily recognize an acoustic neuroma. For example, improved technology can now allow us to see a tumor earlier in its development – even when the neuroma is millimeters in size[20] – whereas that same tumor 50 years ago may have gone unnoticed until many years later when it had grown to a substantial size (and caused substantial problems!). Similarly, access to medical technology has been shown to influence one's likelihood of discovering an acoustic neuroma. To illustrate this, a study from 2006 found that the incidence of acoustic neuroma in Beverly Hills reached 1 in 20,000[21]. The authors of that study suggested one reason for the much higher incidence rate was that the population in Beverly Hills on average had a greater access to medical care, and as such were more likely to be diagnosed.

While advancements in technology can be expected to continue to improve our ability to detect acoustic neuromas, one caveat to further improvements in technology is that the prevalence and incidence of acoustic neuroma are most likely going to continue to increase over time as we become more adept at finding existing tumors. Therefore, we must be careful to separate out whether acoustic neuroma is actually occurring more frequently, or if we are just becoming more adept at finding cases that already exist. If the latter is the issue, then the disease is not truly occurring more frequently; instead, technology simply allows us to find the disease earlier in its development. What we should also expect to happen with earlier diagnosis is that data regarding the age at which an individual is diagnosed with acoustic neuroma begins to decrease, as well as the fact that tumor size at diagnosis will likely be smaller than in prior years. Because the information outlining an increased incidence for acoustic neuroma could be due simply to advancements in diagnostic technology, such change should be acceptable and even encouraged, as it can help us identify affected individuals earlier in the development of acoustic neuroma. Still, we must be careful to not be complacent and continue to investigate whether in fact the disease is indeed occurring more frequently.

Besides overall incidence rates, there are other ways to look at one's chance of developing an acoustic neuroma. For example one study found that from 2004 to 2010, a total of 23,739 acoustic neuromas were diagnosed[22] in the United States. This indicates that an average of around 3,300 new cases of acoustic neuroma occur per year. Similarly, it has been reported that a single individual's risk of developing an acoustic neuroma at any point in their lifetime lies at around 1 in 1000[20]. Along these lines, a separate study reported an occurrence rate of one acoustic neuroma per 100,000 person-years[15]. Person-years is similar to the concept of 'man hours', where if 40 people worked for one hour, an equivalent of 40 'man hours' would have been accomplished. Therefore, one acoustic neuroma per 100,000 person-years means that for every 100,000 years that a group of people accumulate in age, one acoustic neuroma is expected to develop.

# Demographics

Demographics of a condition outline the type of individual who is affected. Examples of what is meant by "type of individual" might include gender, age, ethnicity, or country of origin. For acoustic neuroma, the condition most often affects individuals who fall into the age range of 45-64, while those least affected are aged 0-19 years[15]. Along those lines, only around 15% of acoustic neuromas occur in individuals less than 30 years of age[17]. Therefore, amongst children and the very young, acoustic neuroma is quite rare[17]. In fact, one study reported that the incidence in 0-19 year olds was just 0.05 new cases per 100,000 people, or approximately one case for every 2,000,000 people in that age group. In contrast, amongst the 65-74 year age group there were almost 3 cases per 100,000 people[22].

Gender-specific analysis reveals that there is no real difference in occurrence of acoustic neuroma between women and men when looked at across all age groups, including children[23]. However, specific age ranges can differ in terms of rates of acoustic neuroma occurrence. For example, in the age range of 35-54 years, women are affected slightly more often than males, while in the 65-84 year age group, males had a slightly higher occurrence rate[22]. And although there is a similar occurrence rate of acoustic neuroma between males and females[15], males tend to develop acoustic neuroma at an earlier age (36-42 years) than females (42-56)[24].

Specific to occurrence by ethnicity, the highest percentage of acoustic neuroma (among all possible tumor types) occurs in India, where the rate has been shown to reach 10.6%[25]. This exceeds the rate found in China (10.2%)[26] as well as both England (4.9%)[27] and the United States (4%)[28]. Interestingly, blacks from the African nations of Kenya, Nigeria, and Zimbabwe report the lowest rate (0.5-2.5%) of acoustic neuroma tumors, even lower than their white counterparts (3.7%)[17].

It should be noted that most of the medical literature outlining these specific ethnicity-based occurrence rates is quite old. Given that the incidence rate of acoustic neuroma has been shown to be climbing over the past couple of decades, it would be relevant to update this data so as to account for the improvements in technology that allow for better and earlier diagnosis.

## Acoustic neuroma size

Acoustic neuromas are small bulbous masses that can reach several centimeters across. In discussing the size of an acoustic neuroma, it is generally outlined in terms of its size at the time it is discovered. Speaking in these terms, with the technology we have available at present, an acoustic neuroma can reach anywhere from 1 mm to multiple centimeters-wide[29, 30]. Because the neuroma may continue to grow, establishing a 'diagnostic' size (i.e. the size of the tumor at discovery) can then provide a baseline against which to compare future measurements that will be used to determine whether the neuroma is indeed growing. But in terms of size of an individual tumor, one study did report that there is a downward trend of patients who are found to have larger-sized tumors[19]. These findings, however, may be due to what we just discussed specific to medicine's ability to find tumors at an earlier stage, which simply means that the tumor will not have grown to as large of a size at diagnosis as might have happened in an earlier time.

There is some evidence that symptoms of acoustic neuroma can be dependent upon tumor size, as one study showed that larger tumors are associated with an abnormal walking pattern, facial weakness or abnormal facial sensation, and headache[19]. Similarly, the presence of tinnitus has been shown to be directly associated with tumor size, as was the type of hearing loss experienced (progressive, sudden, fluctuant, or nil)[31]. It has also been shown that patients who have a currently growing tumor also have a higher rate of tinnitus and balance issues[32]. This in turn led the authors of that study to suggest that those symptoms may be related to *growth* of a tumor rather than the mere size of an existing tumor.

Some researchers have suggested that a tumor's size at diagnosis can help predict its likelihood for future growth. For example, it has been reported that larger tumors discovered at diagnosis tend to show less likelihood to grow[33]. However, this finding has been challenged by evidence that patients with larger tumors are at greater risk for tumor growth, and that the presence of tinnitus increases by three times the chance that the tumor will grow[34].

## Acoustic neuroma growth rate

As we discussed, the point at which an acoustic neuroma is discovered is the point at which its size is determined. For example, a neuroma discovered in its early stages will likely be quite small, while a neuroma that has went undiscovered could be expected to have reached a substantial size. Size of an acoustic neuroma is not always a priority, particularly in the case of smaller tumors. Instead, tumor growth rate is often more of a concern, as smaller tumors that continue to grow are likely to end up causing a problem once they reach a certain size.

Generally speaking, acoustic neuromas are considered slow-growing tumors[17]. The norm for growth rate of most acoustic neuromas is from 2-4mm per year[35]. Elderly patients have been reported to experience a much slower growth rate (i.e. 1.4mm/year) than younger populations[36], though other studies have reported no correlation between tumor growth rate and age[37, 38].

Establishing the growth rate of an acoustic neuroma can be somewhat problematic given that they often take on an irregular shape[20] that is somewhat due to the fact that they grow in a confined area that can result in their being compressed by other structures. For example, the internal acoustic meatus (IAC), that bony tunnel which runs through the skull and allows the facial and vestibulocochlear nerve to pass from the ear to the brain, is a common location for an acoustic neuroma to first form. Because the IAC is bone, the softer tumor cannot simply push the bone out of the way like it can other structures; therefore, the tumor tends to grow to the point that it assumes the shape of the IAC interior before expanding outward to the soft environment of the brain cavity. Once reaching the brain cavity the neuroma can then expand in size without much resistance. The resulting variation in shape can lead to difficulty in measuring the true size of the acoustic neuroma. Furthermore, inconsistencies in how acoustic neuromas are measured from one research study to the next limits the ability to compare growth rates of these tumors across large sets of data as is commonly done in the research literature[20].

Because of the inherent difficulty in measuring the growth rate of an irregularly-shaped tumor, some researchers prefer to determine growth rate as the time it takes for the acoustic neuroma to double in volume[39]. When using this parameter, the time frame required for a tumor to double in size has been shown to take anywhere from 1.65 to 4.4 years, highlighting the wide range of growth rates that occur with this type of neuroma.

*Expected acoustic neuroma growth*

Few would argue that growth of an acoustic neuroma can be problematic, and any tumor that continues to grow will almost certainly cause problems for a patient down the road. Unfortunately, there has yet to be a clear factor identified that would allow us to predict a tumor's growth rate[20]. Theories as to what can affect growth rate have been proposed, such as molecular composition of the tumor[20], but as of yet a true trigger for what initiates tumor growth has yet to be identified. Instead, we are left with patterns that have been established specific to growth of an acoustic neuroma including phases of no growth, initial growth followed by non-growth, initial growth followed by regression (i.e.

'shrinkage'), continuous regression, or continuous growth[40].

The research has long made clear this inconsistency that is inherent to acoustic neuroma growth. For example, it has been reported that an acoustic neuroma exhibiting minimal to no growth over a 1.5-3 year period will most likely not grow to any significant size[41]. However, in holding consistent with the unpredictability of acoustic neuroma growth, research has found contradictory evidence to this such that some acoustic neuromas do in fact grow after a period of zero growth[38]. Similarly, patients with an initially non-growing tumor were found to have small increments of growth (i.e. 1/2 centimeter) over subsequent years[42]. And more recent evidence collected on over 500 patients recognizes that growth of an acoustic neuroma does occur, yet this growth typically ceases within five years of diagnosis[38]. This finding was similar to that found in a broader study that reviewed the available research showing that around 50% of acoustic neuromas showed no growth during the period of observation, approximately 40-45% did indeed grow, and 6-8% shrunk in size[20].

Outlining this growth rate information is important, as growth of an acoustic neuroma has increasingly become the determining factor behind whether intervention is required or whether the tumor will continue to be monitored, particularly among small to medium sized neuromas[20]. For example, conservative treatment has become an emerging option for patients. Even for neuromas that received no medical intervention at all (i.e. conservative treatment), 40% have been shown to not exhibit any continued growth after diagnosis. Furthermore, up to 10% of neuromas decrease in size per year[35]. This is not to say that conservative treatment is preferred, though, as a separate study did show that in the 10 years following diagnosis, most patients can expect to experience *some* degree of tumor growth[39], with anywhere from 30-90% of neuromas expected to increase in size[38].

It is also important to note that some reports have indicated that growth rate of a tumor can influence the patient's associated symptoms – such as that of disequilibrium and imbalance[43] as well as hearing[44]. One report even linked tumor growth rate with long-term hearing retainment, as the authors found that if an acoustic neuroma grows less than or equal to 2.5mm per year, patients tended to have better hearing over time[44]. But this is also not guaranteed, as patients may still lose their hearing over time, even when the acoustic neuroma appears to have had no change in size[45]. Similarly, research has suggested a relationship between tumor growth and hearing loss, as a growth rate of more than 2.5mm per year can be indicative of future hearing loss[46].

When stepping back and looking at all of the growth-related research, the collective findings indicate that an acoustic neuroma can quite simply grow, shrink, or remain the same size[38].  Stated more bluntly, growth of acoustic neuroma is quite unpredictable.

## Continuously-growing neuromas

Fortunately, neuromas that grow continuously (i.e. without stopping) are less common, consisting of only around 15-25% of tumors studied[20].  Among tumors that do continue to grow, the growth rate can reach 2-4mm per year, though up to 15% of tumors can grow more than 1 centimeter (cm) per year[47].  In some extremely rare cases, a growth rate of nearly 20mm per year has occurred[20].

## True growth vs. treatment-induced growth

It is important to establish whether growth observed in an acoustic neuroma is due to a natural cause (i.e. increase in overall tissue mass) or ancillary to some other factor.  For example, even after radiation a large acoustic neuroma may experience additional – though temporary – growth as a result of radiation-induced swelling[48].  In such cases, the tumor is not growing due to an increase in tissue mass but rather due to the swelling brought on by the strenuous radiation treatment it has endured.

# Cause of Acoustic Neuroma

One of the main questions that researchers still want to know is *what causes acoustic neuroma?* While it would certainly be beneficial to have an established cause for acoustic neuroma, unfortunately the science available at this time can't provide an answer. However, we do have insight into factors that increase one's risk of developing an acoustic neuroma, and those risks could potentially lend evidence to help establish a cause. For example, research initially pointed to noise exposure as a risk factor for acoustic neuroma, as men working in loud-noise environments for 20 or more years were twice as likely to develop acoustic neuroma compared to those who did not have a job in which they were exposed to loud noise[49]. While this evidence of an increased risk could be expected to lead to directed efforts to find out *why* noise levels may trigger an acoustic neuroma, later research did not reach a similar finding specific to loud noise increasing one's risk for developing acoustic neuroma[50]. As such, more research must be conducted in order to better identify loud noise as a possible trigger for acoustic neuroma.

## *Medical history*

A person's medical history may lend clues specific to their risk potential for developing an acoustic neuroma. For example, one study reported that individuals with a history of hay fever were at increased risk of developing an acoustic neuroma[50]. However, a link outlining why hay fever and acoustic neuroma are linked was not established, and as such this report remains only an association between two factors rather than a true cause. Interestingly, the same study revealed that patients with a history of cancer in their family appeared to be at increased risk, but once those patients' employment settings were factored in, those same patients' risk for developing an acoustic neuroma decreased to the point that it lost its association with employment. This may be due to the fact that certain employment settings can offer better health care, which in turn leads to improved diagnosis and/or treatment options for acoustic neuroma[50].

Because we are discussing potential causes of acoustic neuroma, we have to also consider the link between acoustic neuroma and neurofibromatosis (NF). Neurofibromatosis is a genetic disease that influences nerve growth and development, and as a disease affects approximately 1 in every 3000 individuals[51]. Consequently, the abnormal tissue growth associated with acoustic neuroma is linked to NF. Subtypes of NF include NF-2, which affects approximately 1 in 25,000 individuals and is specific to acoustic neuroma itself. Research has shown that acoustic neuromas are linked to the NF-2 gene, specifically what the gene codes for – a protein known as moesin-ezrin-radixin-like protein, or "merlin"[52]. Merlin serves to suppress tumors (among other functions); therefore, a faulty merlin gene – or inactivation of that gene[13]) – can allow for the development of an acoustic neuroma[52]. Merlin's role in tumor suppression and the specificity between NF2 and acoustic neuroma have led to NF-2 being a suspected culprit behind acoustic neuroma.

*Nerve tissue involvement*

As we have discussed, the vestibular nerve is the structure from which an acoustic neuroma first originates. If you remember back to the previous chapter, we discussed nerve myelination, including that point during a nerve's growth in which its development transitions from nerve tissue to myelinated tissue. Acoustic neuroma is suspected to arise from this transition zone within the nerve's outermost cells, a point at which the cells of the nerve sheath (i.e. "glial" cells) transition over to Schwann cells[17]. It remains unknown as to why an acoustic neuroma occurs within this area, but one theory is that this transition area contains a high amount of 'precursor' Schwann cells, or cells that have not yet differentiated into the actual Schwann cell[53]. It's possible that some as-yet-undiscovered mechanism triggers these precursor cells to grow – and in some cases grow unregulated – which we in turn would recognize as an acoustic neuroma. Still, much research remains to be done to establish these precursor cells as the definitive cause of acoustic neuroma.

# Symptoms of Acoustic Neuroma

In many cases, acoustic neuroma patients are found to have a relatively small tumor which triggers minimal symptoms and causes little if any disruption to their normal activities[54]. Because acoustic neuromas grow within the skull and are themselves quite slow-growing, there is not often a significant event that triggers a patient to seek medical attention. In contrast, other vestibular conditions such as Ménière's disease or vestibular migraine often elicit a sudden and violent bout of headache or vertigo that can often end up with the patient making a trip to the emergency room.

With the advent of technology that can now recognize tumors of 1mm or less, the associated symptoms in these small tumors at the time of diagnosis may be quite mild. The truly problematic symptoms of acoustic neuroma such as disabling neurological complications do not typically occur in acoustic neuromas smaller than 30mm[55]. Therefore, it is imperative that acoustic neuroma patients who do seek medical attention provide as much detail about their symptoms as possible. This can help ensure that their medical professional has a complete set of information and that proper care can be administered to help prevent the more debilitating effects.

For patients with an existing acoustic neuroma, the most common symptoms include hearing loss on the affected side in 96% of patients, balance issues in around

77%, and tinnitus within 71%[17]. Unfortunately, these three main symptoms are also quite common in the general population and can often, as in the case of hearing loss, be associated with the normal aging process. As such, it is not uncommon for an individual who is experiencing a low-level of hearing loss or perhaps slight unsteadiness to dismiss the symptoms as simply 'getting old'. And the evidence backs up this idea, as only about 10% of patients who exhibit these symptoms are found to indeed have an acoustic neuroma. However, one-sided hearing loss is almost always the first symptom of acoustic neuroma[56], and the fact that the hearing loss occurs on one side should help separate acoustic-neuroma-associated hearing loss from normal age-associated hearing loss. Notably, the average time frame between one-sided hearing loss and diagnosis of acoustic neuroma ranges from 1-3 years, indicating that it is not uncommon for patients to wait a significant amount of time before seeking treatment, even though symptoms like hearing loss are evident.

In addition to hearing loss, balance issues, and tinnitus, acoustic neuroma patients also report issues such as headache in 29% of patients, ear/jaw pain in 28%, facial numbness (7%), and double-vision (7%)[57]. It is important to note that these symptoms and all symptoms of acoustic neuroma share some similarity with other vestibular disorders such as vestibular migraine (See Chapter 6). Therefore, it is imperative that an individual experiencing any of these symptoms gets evaluated by a medical professional in order to receive a thorough evaluation of those structures capable of causing the symptoms. And, reports are conflicting as to whether symptoms are related to tumor size[31, 58]; therefore, a person experiencing one-sided hearing loss in conjunction with tinnitus could have a rather small tumor within their ear just the same as they could be experiencing a larger acoustic neuroma or even no tumor at all.

It is also important to note that the location of the acoustic neuroma within the inner ear can influence its symptoms. Most often, acoustic neuromas form within the internal acoustic meatus of the temporal bone[59] that allows the vestibulocochlear and facial nerves to pass from the inner ear to the brain. When located within this structure, acoustic neuromas are described as intracanalicular, or 'within the canal'. If the neuroma proceeds to stick out of the canal, it is termed an extracanalicular neuroma. When the acoustic neuroma does become extracanalicular it can have effects on other structures besides the vestibulocochlear and facial nerve. For example, it can compress other cranial nerves as well as the brainstem or the cerebellum[59]. Those tumors located outside of the internal acoustic meatus are more likely to grow and trigger additional symptoms than tumors located within the canal[38].

The length of time that symptoms exist prior to being diagnosed with acoustic neuroma has been reported to average around 18 months, though there can be quite a wide range in this timeframe[60]. No matter the length of time an individual has exhibited symptoms, it must be pointed out that treating the symptoms directly will most likely have no effect, as acoustic neuroma symptoms tend to maintain a presence despite directed treatment[32]. Therefore, symptom relief should be largely focused on treatment of the acoustic neuroma (i.e. the cause of the symptoms) rather than treating specific symptoms. Now, we'll take an in-depth look at some of the more common symptoms associated with acoustic neuroma.

*Hearing loss*

As discussed, hearing loss in one ear is the most common initial symptom of acoustic neuroma. Hearing loss is thought to occur due to the tumor compressing either the vestibulocochlear nerve or the nerve's blood supply[61]. The degree of hearing loss resulting from acoustic neuroma is most often gradual over time but can in some cases (10-20%) be sudden[62]. This is important for patients to be aware of, as acoustic neuroma patients with slowly progressing hearing loss as their initial symptom tend to have slower tumor growth than patients with sudden hearing loss, tinnitus, or dizziness[40]. But it is also important to keep hearing loss in context – even when sudden in nature – as only about 1% of those with sudden hearing loss are found to have an acoustic neuroma[63]. This 1% though, may change over time with improved ability (e.g. more sensitive MRI) to detect those tumors that are capable of causing sudden hearing loss.

When it comes to acoustic neuroma diagnosis, around 95% of patients will have experienced hearing loss in conjunction with their neuroma. In other words, only about 5% will present with normal hearing at diagnosis. Those patients with normal hearing or low-frequency loss of hearing have been associated with a small tumor[64]. Patients with mid- to high-frequency hearing loss were more likely to have a medium-sized tumor, while patients with extensive hearing loss or deafness were most often found to have a large tumor[64]. It is suspected that as the tumor grows, it compresses the nearby cochlear nerve, in turn reducing the ability of that nerve to transmit signals from the cochlea to the brain[64].

The degree of hearing loss does not depend solely on the size of the acoustic neuroma; therefore, hearing loss is not likely due solely to compression of the cochlear nerve[65]. If it were true that hearing loss was proportional to the size of a patient's neuroma, then it would be logical to suspect that as a tumor increases in size, the ability of the cochlear nerve to transmit signals would be diminished. But this argument falls flat, as larger acoustic neuromas are not consistently found in patients with the highest degree of hearing loss. Still, there is evidence that an association does exist between acoustic neuroma and hearing loss given that acoustic neuroma has been shown to cause a greater loss of inner ear hair cells[66]. Given that these hair cells have an important role in our ability to hear, such loss of these hair cells would explain diminished hearing in some acoustic neuroma patients even when the cochlear nerve is not compressed.

While cochlear nerve compression and hair cell loss are viable explanations for diminished hearing on the same side as the tumor, several other suggested causes for hearing loss have been proposed. These causes include endolymphatic hydrops, metabolic abnormalities, alteration of inner ear fluid composition, and reduced action of the stapes bone[67]. While each has a viable physiological rationale as to how it could contribute to hearing loss, the fact remains that we just don't know the true cause behind the hearing loss, leading to the evident point that more research is needed in order to establish which event(s) truly contribute to the cause for hearing loss.

While hearing loss is a common symptom of acoustic neuroma, even one-sided hearing loss does not always indicate the presence of an acoustic neuroma. Still, other ear-related events can influence the chance of receiving an acoustic neuroma diagnosis. For example, some cases have shown that if a patient reports diminished hearing after a certain event (e.g. gunfire), it can increase the chance that an acoustic neuroma is missed during the subsequent evaluation[17]. Similarly, if another condition or symptom such as tinnitus also exists – or if the patient's symptoms are unique from the more commonly reported symptoms of acoustic neuroma – the neuroma itself is more likely to be missed during the evaluation.

*Vertigo and balance issues*

Because acoustic neuromas arise from the vestibular nerve, it is not uncommon for patients to experience some degree of balance issues and/or vertigo. In fact, disequilibrium has been reported in 40% of acoustic neuroma patients, vertigo in 28%, and dizziness in 22%.

Typically, patients report some degree of these imbalance issues for years prior to diagnosis; therefore, a sudden onset of vertigo or unsteadiness is not typical of acoustic neuroma[17]. Although the acoustic neuroma does arise directly from the vestibular nerve, its slow growth rate explains the expected slow onset of imbalance issues. In addition, the fact that the opposite vestibular nerve is typically intact in cases of acoustic neuroma can explain why the patient is not severely affected by imbalance in most cases[17]. Elderly patients, however, are most susceptible to exhibiting more pronounced effects of imbalance[17]. And nausea – often associated with vertigo and found in multiple other vestibular disorders such as Ménière's disease – does not typically occur with instability relating to acoustic neuroma[17].

## Tinnitus

Tinnitus is the perception of sound when no sound actually exists. For acoustic neuroma patients, tinnitus has been reported as one of the most frustrating symptoms associated with the condition[68]. In one study, 60% of patients with a known acoustic neuroma reported tinnitus[69]. Typically, the tinnitus is thought to arise from a source other than the area of the tumor itself[68], leading to the likelihood that the tumor is not directly responsible for the tinnitus but does contribute to its presence.

Tinnitus associated with acoustic neuroma is most often constant in nature and noticeable only in the affected ear, though the type of perceived sound (i.e. high-pitch, low hum, whistle, etc.) is not consistent among patients[17]. Unfortunately, even severing of the cochlear portion of the vestibulocochlear nerve during surgical treatment for neuroma does not alleviate the tinnitus in up to 37% of patients[70]. Therefore, treatment decisions are not recommended to be focused on an attempt to alleviate tinnitus[68] but should instead remain geared toward treating the neuroma itself or other significant symptoms.

## Ataxia

The condition of ataxia involves an appearance of being 'drunk' – slurred speech, imbalance, stumbling or tripping often, and uncoordinated muscle movements.

Most often, ataxia results from an underlying neural condition that is ultimately revealed after investigating these various symptoms.

When acoustic neuroma is the cause of ataxia, it is typically the result of a severe case such as the tumor being of significant size to compress the cerebellum area of the brain[17]. The cerebellum plays a major role in muscle coordination, so any compression of the cerebellum could be expected to impact normal muscle function in the body. Along these lines, some acoustic neuroma patients have been shown to lean towards the side of the tumor as a result of cerebellum compression[17]. In some cases, the brain stem may also be compressed[17].

## Conclusion

While our understanding of acoustic neuroma has improved greatly, there is still much that we need to learn. Aspects such as why the tumor occurs, what causes it to change in size, and what factors can predict its course are all areas that need further investigation. Still, the outcome of acoustic neuroma has changed immensely from those unfortunate early years as research and improvements in technology have allowed for earlier diagnosis and more precise identification of the neuroma. Next, we'll take a look at the equipment and techniques commonly used in the diagnosis of acoustic neuroma in order to provide you an overview of the steps that physicians and other medical professionals use in recognizing the neuroma.

# Chapter 3 – Diagnosis

Diagnosis is the process of establishing whether or not and individual has a disease. As a patient, physicians and other medical professionals arrive at a diagnosis after evaluating a collection of information that includes your medical history, your symptoms, and the results of a set of medical tests that they order. Most likely, you visited your physician due to symptoms that you felt were unusual, and at some point those symptoms either hadn't gone away or you felt that they were significant enough that you needed a medical professional's opinion. Prior to your final diagnosis, it's likely that you had to visit multiple professionals due to your symptoms not falling within a particular physician's specialty, and he or she felt that another type of physician would better serve your needs. Or perhaps you desired to seek a second opinion on your own to get a clearer understanding of your situation. Either way, having multiple physician visits likely subjected you to a range of medical tests and procedures, and at some point you may have wondered what all was occurring on your journey toward a diagnosis.

It is important to know that every test performed on you served to provide your physician a key piece of information that he or she could piece together to arrive at a final diagnosis. Eventually, a diagnosis was indeed reached that established your condition as acoustic neuroma. In order to help you understand the steps involved in diagnosis of acoustic neuroma, this chapter is focused on providing you an overview of the various tests and associated parameters that allow medical professionals to determine that you have an acoustic neuroma. We will not cover all possible tests in this chapter, as there are many tests out there and not every medical professional uses every test. Rather, we will focus on those that are commonly used in and provide the most beneficial information for the diagnosis of acoustic neuroma.

## Classifying an acoustic neuroma

Though suffering through the symptoms associated with acoustic neuroma is by no means an enjoyable experience, one favorable aspect is that the culprit – i.e. the tumor itself – can be visualized through several available imaging techniques such as computerized tomography (CT) scanning or magnetic resonance imaging (MRI). Other inner ear conditions such as Ménière's disease or vestibular migraine bring on similar symptoms of imbalance or hearing loss yet have no recognizable physical mass to aid professionals in diagnosing the condition. As such, diagnosis of those other conditions often occurs after ruling all other medical conditions out, including acoustic neuroma. With the presence of an acoustic neuroma, however, imaging techniques make it possible to identify the physical structure of the tumor. When it's in the right place and combined with a few specific symptoms, a diagnosis of acoustic neuroma can be relatively simple to establish.

As we discussed in the prior chapter, acoustic neuromas arise from the vestibular nerve and grow to various, unpredictable sizes. Often, the tumor is simply described by its size in millimeters or centimeters. Obviously, overall size of the tumor plays a role in the potential severity of the tumor, particularly within the confined area of the skull. As yet, though, there is no system that exists which classifies an acoustic neuroma according to factors such as risk to the patient, ranking tumors by severity, or similar. Instead, a classification system that has been around since 1976 is still used to outline the various stages of an acoustic neuroma, though these stages are based only upon tumor location and size rather than tumor severity or risk. This classification, known as the *Koos classification system,* is as follows[71]:

Stage 1: Intra-canalicular tumor (diameter 1-10mm)
Stage 2: Tumor extends beyond internal acoustic

meatus (diameter less than 20mm)

Stage 3:  Tumor extends into cerebellopontine angle but
             does not compress the brainstem (diameter less
             than 30mm)

Stage 4:  Tumor causing brainstem compression
             (diameter greater than 30mm)

While the Koos classification system is based somewhat upon the neuroma's reference to certain anatomical structures, acoustic neuroma is to some degree still predominantly classified based upon its diameter. With the advanced imaging technology available in this day and age we can often diagnose smaller tumors at an earlier stage than have been recognized previously. Given the similarity in symptoms between acoustic neuroma and several other inner-ear conditions, proper diagnosis of the tumor is key to reducing the potential for misdiagnosis of conditions such as noise-induced hearing loss, age-related hearing loss, tinnitus, vestibulopathy, Ménière's disease, or sudden deafness with vertigo, rather than acoustic neuroma[60].

# Medical history

We outlined in the past chapter how medical history can provide key bits of information as to one's risk of having an acoustic neuroma. Medical history can also play a predominant role in diagnosis. During the initial physician visit, the patient should provide as much relevant information as possible specific to what brought him or her to seek medical attention. Symptoms, events, and anything that could be related to their current medical state should be discussed with the physician. For example, if a patient's mother or father has had lifelong dizziness, that would certainly be relevant for a patient to discuss during their visit. Or if there has been persistent tinnitus that started for no reason, or if the hearing has diminished in one ear more than another, those aspects should be outlined in the patient's discussion of their medical history.

One important thing to remember about medical history is that it is highly subjective. This means that the patient must provide the information while the physician listens to and processes that same information. For example, if a patient says he or she has developed a ringing sound in their ear, there is no currently available test that can measure the degree of tinnitus they are experiencing. Instead, the patient must take the time to point out that the tinnitus affects their ability to sleep, impacts normal conversation, and perhaps causes a significant degree of anxiety. And, if the tinnitus is only in one ear, that is of significance and should be reported as well. Other relevant points might include siblings or parents with a similar condition, workplace noise levels, medication taken, and any disabling aspects (e.g. reduced ability to hear conversation in noisy environments). The more information that a patient can provide, the better a physician can start to piece together a diagnosis that is built off of material provided by the patient.

## Imaging

As hinted at previously, the advent of certain medical imaging devices has been a godsend of sorts for inner-ear patients. Now, rather than undergoing exploratory surgery to determine the source of a problem, a clearly-defined and precisely-located tumor can be identified in the time it takes to obtain and read an MRI scan. This is certainly much more advantageous than the early process of undergoing a risky, highly invasive surgical procedure just to see if a neuroma is indeed present. To highlight some of the available technology, we'll next take a look at the most commonly used imaging techniques in order to outline their application in the diagnosis of acoustic neuroma.

### Computed Tomography scan

The use of computed tomography (CT) has been around for decades. Think of CT as a 3-dimensional x-ray, as several x-rays are taken in succession and then 'stacked' into one image that is then presented 3-dimensionally. The procedure is convenient, simple, and quick, and can play an important role in the diagnosis of acoustic neuroma.

One of the benefits of CT scanning for acoustic neuroma is that large tumors can typically be detected via CT[13]. Unfortunately, smaller tumors are more likely to be missed[13]. Image analysis in acoustic neuroma identification has also shown that CT is particularly beneficial for outlining the local bony anatomy around the acoustic neuroma such as expansion of the diameter of the internal auditory canal that can occur with more aggressive neuromas[13].

*Magnetic Resonance Imaging*

Over the years, magnetic resonance imaging (MRI) has grown to become the gold standard for evaluating and monitoring acoustic neuromas[13]. These days, when an acoustic neuroma is suspected, it is not uncommon for the patient to be sent for an MRI given how the scan can reveal much about tumor size and shape (Figure 3.1). In addition, an MRI can be helpful in planning out the most appropriate treatments for a particular tumor[13]. While the MRI is typically more expensive and takes longer than a CT scan, the results are much more detailed for acoustic neuroma detections.

With its sensitive technology, the MRI scan can show an enhanced image of the acoustic neuroma, and more than half of acoustic neuromas can appear as clear as surrounding tissue[72]. Because of the sensitivity of the MRI, a scan can even capture events such as bleeding that is occurring within the tumor[13].

When monitoring an acoustic neuroma over time to check for growth, the detail provided by an MRI allows for precise measurement of tumor size, thereby allowing for detailed analysis into whether tumor growth is occurring[73]. In fact, when used in conjunction with a particular dye called gadolinium, MRI can detect an acoustic neuroma less than $0.05cm^3$ in size[30]. Remember last chapter when we mentioned that the incidence rate of acoustic neuroma is increasing? The improvement of imaging technology such as the MRI has likely played a significant role in this increase, as smaller tumors were not detectable with technology that existed prior to the MRI.

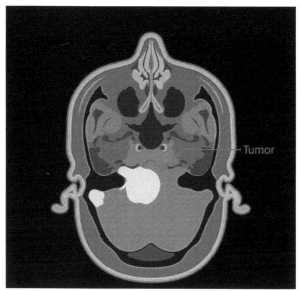

*Figure 3.1. A representation of how a large acoustic neuroma appears similar to a white ball on MRI*

# Ear function

Whereas a reduction in hearing is a common complaint with acoustic neuroma, physicians will often order a set of tests to evaluate aspects such as hearing and inner-ear function. Such tests often include an audiogram as well as speech or sound discrimination[72], both of which are outlined below. The particular tests ordered are often dependent upon each patient's reported symptoms, as patients who report hearing loss would be expected to undergo a hearing evaluation while those with balance issues will likely be subjected to vestibular testing[59]. Now we'll discuss some of these ear-function tests that are used to evaluate acoustic neuroma in order to gain a better understanding of how the information derived from these tests aids medical professionals in diagnosis.

*Audiogram*

The measurement of whether an individual's hearing has been affected by an acoustic neuroma is dependent upon the results of a hearing test, or "audiogram". Besides imaging of the inner ear such as through MRI, one of the initial tests that many medical professionals order is the audiogram to determine the patient's ability to hear sound (Figure 3.2). Because hearing loss is one of the first symptoms of acoustic neuroma, the audiogram can provide valuable data as to

81

the likelihood of an existing tumor[72]. The process of measuring the individual's hearing is known as pure-tone audiometry. For acoustic neuroma patients, a loss of high-frequency tones is one of the most common hearing-related issues[56].

Conducting an audiogram consist of two main aspects – performing the test itself and analyzing the graph. To perform the test, the patient wears headphones and is subjected to a range of tones delivered at specific levels, or "Hertz" (Hz). The patient then indicates when he or she hears those sounds, and the lowest sound heard by the patient at each level is then recorded on a graph. Though results can vary from patient to patient, findings from the audiogram typically involve tone, decay in hearing, and an absence of recruitment[56].

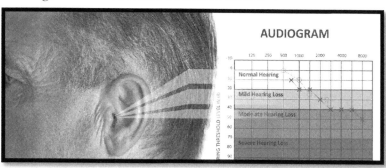

Figure 3.2  The audiogram is a plot of a patient's ability to hear sounds at certain frequencies.

## Caloric testing

Long ago, it was revealed that putting cool and warm water or air into the ear canal, or 'caloric testing' (the word *caloric* means 'heat') could elicit a certain response within the inner ear. Prior to our modern imaging technology, the caloric procedure was reported to be the best test for recognizing larger tumors, though it was not as reliable with smaller tumors[74]. It was also long considered a beneficial test for establishing the likely presence of an acoustic neuroma as the test has been shown to be 'normal' in less than 4% of acoustic neuroma patients[75].

The caloric test is particularly useful in stimulating the horizontal semicircular canal which sends signals along the superior portion of the vestibular nerve[67]. A positive caloric test in such a case typically indicates that the tumor exists on the superior portion of the vestibular nerve, while a normal (i.e. 'negative') caloric test often indicates that the tumor is on the inferior portion of the nerve[76]. Similarly, a normal caloric test is often associated with good hearing preservation as well as a high likelihood for normal facial nerve function after surgery[77]. There is also some degree of tumor size revealed by the caloric test, as tumors are typically larger in patients with a positive caloric test while patients with smaller tumors commonly have normal caloric tests[78].

The caloric test is sometimes combined with electrodes placed around the patient's eyes. This allows for recording the activity of the eye muscles which in turns makes the caloric test a type of electronystagmography. Unusual eye movements in response to caloric testing can lead to a suspicion of vestibular nerve involvement, thus providing valuable evidence as to the likelihood of an acoustic neuroma.

## Brainstem auditory evoked response

The brainstem auditory evoked response, also known as *brainstem evoked response audiometry* or *auditory brainstem response*, was once considered the preferred diagnostic test for patients suspected of having an acoustic neuroma[67]. Much like caloric testing, however, improvements in diagnostic technology such as the MRI have diminished the need for the brainstem evoked response test.

The test itself is designed to determine whether hearing is able to occur between the ear and the brain stem[72] by measuring brain activity in response to certain sounds (e.g. 'clicks'). As a patient, small electrodes are placed around your forehead and ear lobes, after which a sound-generating device is placed near your ear. At the start of the test, a particular pattern of clicks are heard from the device. The medical professional will then record how fast your brain reacts to these sounds. The degree of brain activity that occurs in response to the sounds is indicative of your ability to process sound.

## Speech discrimination

Speech discrimination testing differs from audiometry in that it is not a measure of sounds in general but instead it tests a patient's ability to understand actual speech. So even though a patient may have the ability to hear sound, the speech discrimination test measures their ability to discern the spoken word. With acoustic neuroma, even when an audiogram is normal an individual's speech discrimination capability can be compromised[79].

To perform the speech discrimination test, the patient simply listens to a series of spoken words at a pre-determined level and then repeats those words back to the medical professional. In addition to 'plain' speech, the speech discrimination test can be modified in order to test other factors. For example, background noise can be introduced with the spoken words heard by the patient. Alternatively, sound can be used to mask the opposite ear so as to limit any perception of sound heard from the opposite (good) ear.

In order to score the test, the medical professional determines to what degree an individual can hear 'normal' speech, then ranks the patient's hearing ability as a percentage. For example, if ranking 100% on the speech discrimination score, this indicates that the patient is able to understand all of the speech patterns presented. Specific to acoustic neuroma and the speech discrimination test, patients who score better than 70% on their test generally maintain good hearing for an average of almost five more years, while two in three patients with a score of 100% tend to continue with good hearing for another 10 years[44].

# Conclusion

Every acoustic neuroma patient is different. Some patients who exhibit particular symptoms can have their diagnosis be a quick, relatively simple process. For other patients, the journey to getting a final diagnosis may require multiple physicians and involve a myriad of diagnostic tests. Regardless of how the patient arrived at their diagnosis, the next phase of life with acoustic neuroma then begins as they enter the treatment phase. A treatment plan must then be formulated in order to deal with the tumor, and this plan is dependent upon many factors such as tumor size, growth rate, or effect on quality of life. In the next chapter, we'll outline several of the treatment options that range from conservative in nature to highly aggressive. Regardless of the plan, the outcome – improving the patient's ability to live a productive life with acoustic neuroma – remains the same.

# Chapter 4 – Treatment

For most of the typical acoustic neuroma patient's life, they have no reason to suspect that there is a tumor growing within their inner ear. At some point, however, certain symptoms such as an onset of tinnitus or a bout of unsteadiness may convince them to speak with a physician. Once they receive a final diagnosis of acoustic neuroma, their mindset most likely shifts towards how to get rid of it. Thus, the patient has entered into the treatment phase of acoustic neuroma in which a plan is enacted with the intent of helping to improve their situation.

Prior to advances in the treatment of acoustic neuroma, patients were often given two options – a slow and miserable death or a risky, highly-invasive surgery[68]. Even if you survived the surgery, you were typically left with a significant degree of vestibular disability or even facial paralysis. But with the improvements that the acoustic neuroma field has experienced specific to techniques, diagnostic equipment, and treatment, the outlook for patients has improved tremendously. Now, advancements in treatment allow for improved cranial nerve function, a better quality of life, and decreased sickness and death rates[80].

The shift in treatment of acoustic neuroma has been remarkable. What originally left patients with the unfortunate options of either a slow death or significant disability has been replaced by modern-day options that include continued observation of the tumor, multiple surgical techniques, or radiation[81]. And treatment goals have changed as well, as the goal in the early days of acoustic neuroma focused strictly on removal of the tumor. This goal was probably linked to the fact that at the time, diagnosis typically didn't occur until the tumor was quite large and therefore causing significant problems. Now, with improved diagnostic technologies (i.e. CT scan, MRI, etc.), acoustic neuroma can be recognized much earlier. In turn, the preferred outcome has shifted away from planned removal of a tumor and has instead focused more toward monitoring the tumor as long as the patient can maintain normal abilities (e.g. nerve function, hearing, etc.)[13] and a favorable quality of life.

Another major objective in the treatment of acoustic neuroma is to preserve hearing for as long as possible[17]. This goal, however, can be complicated by the fact that hearing-based symptoms often arise in the later stages of the disease[82], thereby indicating that a more aggressive treatment of the tumor (e.g. surgery) may be necessary in order to maintain the patient's hearing status. Along these lines, other factors that can influence the type of treatment to be used with acoustic neuroma include the location of the tumor, the patient's age, other medical issues that a patient may have (i.e. 'comorbidities'), and/or the potential surgical risk to the patient[80].

We certainly did not arrive at our current state of acoustic neuroma treatment easily. When that slow and miserable death was the only option, interventions were attempted that tried to give some degree of improvement, even though the early attempts still resulted in death. But over time, a lot of trial and error along with many well-designed research studies have led us to where we are now, which is undoubtedly a vast improvement from where we started. Still, we have not cured the condition of acoustic neuroma, nor have we developed a flawless treatment plan. As such, more work must be done and more research needs to be conducted. Along those lines, part of the problem that neuroma patients find when it comes to treatment is that there is not a high level of research comparing the various treatment options available[68]. Furthermore, there has been quite a bit of variation in treatment between medical centers as well as between surgeons, and this variation further complicates the ability to compare available options[68].

It is also of interest to note how in treatment of acoustic neuroma, the fact that we have *some* viable options has impacted our ability to continue to conduct effective research. This stems from the fact that patients have been found to be reluctant to allow themselves to be assigned to an unproven treatment when other, known treatments exist[83]. As such it can be difficult to try out potentially beneficial treatments on patients given that they often prefer to stick to more proven treatments with more well-known outcomes.

# Treatment options

Acoustic neuroma patients have three primary choices when it comes to treatment of their tumor – conservative treatment, radiation treatment, or surgery. Now we'll take a look at these three options in order to outline the main components of each and help you understand the theories and indications behind each treatment. It must be pointed out, though, that this chapter is not designed to be a tool to help you decide which treatment is best. Rather, that is a decision that should be made between you and your physician, as he or she will be able to work with you to develop the best treatment option for your particular case.

*Conservative treatment*

Prior to the availability of medical imaging such as CT and MRI that we have available now, almost all tumors were recommended for removal once diagnosed[17]. For larger tumors, this was understandable given the size that the tumors often reached prior to being recognized, as well as the known complications (e.g. hearing loss, imbalance, etc.) that large tumors can cause[17]. Improvements in imaging technology along with our better understanding of the natural course of acoustic neuroma progression has allowed physicians to detect and diagnose much smaller tumors. This in turn has allowed for the development of a 'wait and see' approach that monitors acoustic neuroma growth over time as opposed to using radiation or surgery to eliminate the tumor[84].

Conservative management of acoustic neuroma is generally any treatment that does not involve surgery or use of radiation. Such treatments might include re-imaging the neuroma via MRI or CT scan at specific time intervals (e.g. every 6 months[13]), pharmaceutical intervention[52], or simply working to minimize symptoms. Some researchers have indicated that neuromas 20mm or smaller would benefit from conservative treatment, and that conservative treatment actually works better to preserve facial nerve and hearing function than the more invasive surgery or radiation treatments[85]. Other researchers use 15mm as the point at which they switch from conservative treatment to more active treatment options[86].

One caveat to the conservative approach is that hearing will most likely continue to worsen with conservative treatment[87]. Therefore, if hearing is a priority, the potentially negative outcomes of observation-only treatment must be thoroughly considered[80]. In fact, the evidence indicates that both surgeons and patients are reluctant to remove an acoustic neuroma if there is still a useful degree of hearing in the ear[86]. This has altered some treatment plans such that even larger neuromas may be targeted for long-term observation rather than removal, at least up to that point at which hearing function is lost. Similarly, such a conservative plan also favors those patients who are more concerned about facial nerve function than maintaining hearing in the affected ear[17].

There are two general assumptions that are inherent to pursuing conservative treatment. The first is that the tumor has grown but will not continue to grow further after treatment. The second assumption is that any continued growth will be so slow that it will cause fewer problems for the patient than any invasive treatment would[88]. However, some researchers argue that observation-based treatment ultimately results in further tumor growth and subsequent hearing loss to a greater extent than occurs with early stereotactic radiosurgery[39]. This contradiction outlines the need for more research data in order to establish a clearer understanding of the best treatment outcomes.

In its early days, conservative treatment was largely limited to elderly patients as well as those patients with other significant problems whose life expectancy was expected to be shorter than the timeframe by which the acoustic neuroma would be expected to cause significant problems[89]. Along these lines, some researchers still feel that 'wait and scan' only makes sense for those patients who have a high likelihood of death in the next 5 years, instead preferring radiosurgery as the most viable treatment after tumor diagnosis[39]. Along these same lines, conservative management of acoustic neuroma in a younger population is not always recommended given that tumor growth rates in this age group can be more rapid[17].

*Stereotactic radiosurgery*

Directing a targeted high dose of radiation at the acoustic neuroma is known as stereotactic radiosurgery, alternatively called "gamma knife" surgery. Radiosurgery – along with conservative treatment – has grown in popularity in the United States over the past 20 years[84], a trend reflected in the United Kingdom as well[90]. The suspected reasons for the growth of radiosurgery include the reduced recovery time for the patient, as well as the improved ability for the technique to maintain both facial nerve function and the patient's current state of hearing as compared to a more invasive surgical procedure[91]. In fact, anywhere from 50 – 80% of patients are able to preserve their hearing after radiosurgery[92], with factors including a patient younger than 60 years, an intracanalicular tumor, and a smaller tumor being most favorable for retaining one's hearing[92]. Furthermore, facial nerve function is retained in almost all radiosurgery patients[92].

Researchers have pointed out that there has been quite a bit of misinformation reported about radiosurgery, such as that the procedure will damage a patient's hearing as well as their face, it will cause the tumor to grow, and it will increase one's risk for cancer[92]. These reports, however, have largely been proven false[92].

Much of the available research has compared radiosurgery to traditional surgery given that surgical procedures for acoustic neuroma have been around so long, and likely because there is much less data comparing radiosurgery to the more recent approach of conservative treatment. Determining the success of radiosurgery in comparison to surgery has proven to be somewhat challenging. In fact, the aforementioned study in which patients were reluctant to leave their treatment to chance was based on a comparison of radiosurgery and surgery. That study ultimately failed as a result of an inability to recruit enough patients to be assigned to an experimental group[83]. One study, however, has had success specific to comparing techniques in relation to tumor size. Improved patient outcomes were reported when using radiosurgery over microsurgery on medium-sized tumors[55].

Other research that did not set out to make a direct comparison between radiosurgery and surgery have shown that radiosurgery can deliver favorable outcomes that are comparable to or even better than what has been reported after surgery[59] yet do not incur many of the associated surgical risks such as infection or bleeding[68]. In one study of patients surveyed after either radiosurgery or surgery, a higher level of facial function, reduced eye-related symptoms, and improved functional ability were reported in patients receiving radiosurgery compared to microsurgery[93]. Furthermore, radiosurgery requires no anesthesia[94] or hospitalization[68]. There is also no risk of a condition known as tumor seeding[68], whereby tumor cells become infused with otherwise healthy tissue as a result of the surgical procedures used for acoustic neuroma. Some patients even report that they experience improved hearing after radiosurgery[92, 93] though this is not a predictable or expected outcome of the procedure[94].

Radiosurgery works by applying radiation to the tumor with the intent of halting its growth. When used for the treatment of acoustic neuroma, radiosurgery differs from traditional radiation therapy in that only a single dose of radiation is delivered as opposed to a series of doses[59]. Radiosurgery utilizes multiple beams of radiation focused in a way that the sum of all beams deliver an overall radiation dose to the tumor[59]. The goals of radiosurgery, however, mimic those of traditional radiation therapy in that the intent is still to control and/or halt tumor growth, and radiosurgery has been shown to halt the growth of almost all acoustic neuromas[39]. In addition, radiosurgery also has a primary aim of preserving the function of the affected cranial nerves (e.g. facial nerve) along with getting the patient back to work as soon as possible[95].

## Indications for radiosurgery

There are no specific criteria outlining the use of radiosurgery, though many professionals prefer to utilize it on acoustic neuromas less than 3cm wide[29]. Smaller tumors, those tumors that have arisen after surgery, or neuromas that occur in the elderly are also generally considered as favorable for radiosurgery[80] whereas larger tumors are typically scheduled for traditional surgery[90]. However, in modern times – where very small tumors are often discovered – individuals are more often being recommended for observation as opposed to radiosurgery treatment[94].

## Risks of stereotactic radiosurgery

Radiosurgery is not without its reported shortcomings. It should be noted, however, that many of the negative aspects of radiosurgery are more related to the effects of radiation over time than to the procedure itself[80]. For example, there is an inherent risk that a radiation treatment can turn a tumor from benign to malignant[68]. Estimates for a malignancy resulting from radiosurgery of a benign tumor have ranged from 1 in 1000[96] to 25 in 100,000 cases[97]. As one researcher pointed out, the risk of death from a radiation-induced tumor is irrelevant compared to the low but possible direct risks of surgery[55]. Other researchers have stated that there is in fact no real risk of a tumor turning malignant following radiation surgery[94].

Separately, patients receiving stereotactic radiosurgery typically require a longer follow-up period than patients who undergo surgery[68]. This follow-up is not focused as much on monitoring for potential side effects of the treatment as it is on watching for subsequent tumor growth over time. In other words, the extended follow-up after radiosurgery is needed to observe for treatment effectiveness more than to ensure proper healing from the procedure itself.

Another potential limitation to radiosurgery is that there is a possibility of tissue scarring, which could serve to complicate any future surgery to the area[68]. This in part stems from the possibility that the radiation dose impacts structures located adjacent to the tumor, in turn negatively affecting the function of those structures[59]. For example, the vestibulocochlear nerve, the brainstem, and the cerebellum are all located in close proximity to an acoustic neuroma, and as such could be subject to potential damage from the radiosurgery procedure. The facial nerve and the trigeminal nerve have been reported to be most at risk from radiosurgery; however, the actual occurrence of injury to these structures has decreased in response to lower dosing as well as a more accurate delivery of the radiation[80].

Advancements in imaging technology as well as treatment planning software can provide physicians valuable assistance in outlining precise doses specific to tumor volume that can help reduce the risk of complications[98]. Still, up to 4% of patients can experience facial paralysis with radiosurgery. This paralysis is most often temporary but can in some cases be permanent, particularly when treating larger tumors[99].

Another potential consequence of radiosurgery involves the possibility of reoccurrence of the tumor or even subsequent tumor growth. These events, should they occur, may require additional radiation or even surgery[80]. The risk of tumor regrowth, though, is very low with radiosurgery treatment. One study reported 36 of 100,000 patients had tumor regrowth over 40 years[100] while a separate study found zero regrowth events in 1,142 patients over 15 years[101].

Hearing preservation is also at risk with radiosurgery. Reports indicate that even with successful treatment of the acoustic neuroma, there is often a decline in hearing for months to years following treatment[102]. Current technology has improved the likelihood of preservation of hearing in the majority of acoustic neuroma patients, and facial nerve function is preserved in almost all patients[103]. Compared to patients treated in the early days of radiation therapy, modern-day patients can expect improved hearing outcomes[102], with reports indicating that hearing can be preserved in 60-90% of patients who undergo radiosurgery[39], particularly among those patients with small tumors.

Similar to hearing preservation, greater than 95% of facial and trigeminal nerve function can be maintained after radiosurgery[39]. Such success is largely dependent upon several factors including proper radiation dose, the initial size of the tumor, and overall nerve function prior to surgery[95]. For example, during its initial implementation, radiosurgery tended to use a high dose of radiation which did ultimately decrease the tumor size. However, these higher doses were likely to cause hearing loss as well as facial and trigeminal nerve problems[104]. Because of these risks, it is not uncommon now for radiosurgery to be planned out by an entire team consisting of a neurosurgeon, radiation oncologist, and medical physicist[95].

*Fractionated Radiotherapy*

Similar to stereotactic radiosurgery, where a single radiation dose is given, fractionated radiotherapy involves delivering the radiation over a period of weeks that, when the doses are summed together, is equivalent to one larger dose[59]. This therapy option requires anywhere from 3-30 treatments over a period of weeks[39]. Fractionated radiotherapy allows for surrounding tissue to have a chance to heal between doses while the tumor continues to receive a direct, repetitive dose[59].

Unfortunately, fractionated radiotherapy has shown less consistent outcomes than radiotherapy[39].

# Surgical excision

When conservative treatment either fails or is not an option, patients and their medical providers often decide between stereotactic radiosurgery and surgery itself. As we discussed, stereotactic radiosurgery – though much less invasive – may not always be an option for patient such as if the tumor has reached a certain size. In such cases, surgery is often the treatment of choice.

Surgical excision involves the physical removal of the acoustic neuroma; therefore, surgical intervention is considered as the only treatment that offers a cure for acoustic neuroma[72]. As such, the procedures involved in surgery are highly invasive and occur in an extremely sensitive area of the body. Operation time can be lengthy, with one report indicating an average surgical time of 6.5 hours, but up to 12 hours[81]. Consequently, there are several risks inherent to using a surgical approach for removal of an acoustic neuroma. Fortunately, advancements in surgical technique, including improved procedures, specialized training, and even developments in sterilization have allowed us to make tremendous strides in patient success, not to mention a reduction in side effects. Still, there is not yet a clear choice as to which procedure should be used to extract an acoustic neuroma[17]. Rather, factors such as tumor size, degree of hearing loss, experience of the surgeon, and even patient preference should be factored in[17].

There are three main approaches that physicians use for surgical removal of an acoustic neuroma. The name for each approach largely describes the anatomy involved: middle cranial fossa, retro-sigmoid/sub-occipital, or translabyrinthine[80]. As just mentioned, the technique ultimately selected is often dependent upon several factors which include the acoustic neuroma size, its location, patient's level of hearing, and potential complications[80]. For example, the middle cranial fossa procedure is recommended for small tumors located within the internal auditory canal. Larger tumors are often pursued using the retro-sigmoid approach, while the translabyrinthine technique is recommended for larger neuromas when either preservation of hearing is not important or when it is unlikely that hearing can be spared[80]. Each procedure has its own strengths and weaknesses, and it is important that you as the patient discuss all benefits and complications for each procedure with your physician prior to undergoing the surgery. Next, we'll briefly outline each of these procedures, highlighting the rationale behind each as well as the potential complications.

*Middle Cranial Fossa Approach*

Small tumors recommended for removal that have not yet caused a significant effect on a patients hearing, as well as those tumors located within the internal auditory canal, are often pursued using the middle cranial fossa (MCF) technique. This approach, while decreasing in popularity[68], is considered favorable for small tumors located within the internal auditory canal and also creates the lowest risk to the sensitive structures of the inner ear's labyrinth[72]. This procedure has been shown to preserve pre-operative hearing function in half of patients[105], with up to 70% still maintaining a reasonable amount of hearing 5-10 years after surgery[106]. Furthermore, the MCF technique has been shown to have up to a 76% success rate of hearing preservation compared to 47-58% when the retrosigmoid approach is used[91, 107, 108]. Separately, facial nerve function has been shown to be quite salvageable when using the MCF procedure, as 96% of patients who had a tumor 1.5cm or smaller reported normal or near-normal facial nerve function after surgery[109], and 94.5% in a separate study of patients with a tumor less than 1cm[110]. Specific to preservation of hearing function, there has been no difference reported between MCF and the retrosigmoid technique[111].

As with any invasive procedure, there are inherent risks involved with the MCF procedure. Among the most significant complications are cerebrospinal fluid leak, hearing loss, facial nerve damage, and infection[80]. In addition, the MCF requires retraction of the temporal lobe which in turn puts the patient at increased risk for seizure after the operation[68].

102

## Retrosigmoid approach

The retrosigmoid (RS) technique is the most common procedure for the removal of acoustic neuroma[72], especially for tumors that exist within the internal auditory canal[112]. The internal auditory canal is exposed using this procedure, and one of the benefits of this approach is that injury to the structures of the inner ear are largely avoided[72]. Furthermore, the RS technique can be utilized for larger tumors that may not be optimal for the MCF approach as well as for tumors that may be compressing the brainstem, nerves, or blood vessels[80].

One benefit of the RS technique is that when removing smaller tumors, the RS procedure has been reported to preserve hearing in 60% of patients[106]. And along these lines, patients with tumors less than 2cm in size were able to maintain facial function 90% of the time. Unfortunately, the success rate of retaining facial function with RS surgery appears to decrease as tumor size increases. Only around 67% of patients maintained facial nerve function when the tumor was larger than 2cm[113] and 50% for patients with a 4cm tumor[114]. Still, the RS approach is not limited as to how large of a tumor can be removed[68].

Complications of the RS surgical approach are similar to the MCF, but there is less surgical risk to the facial nerve due to its position compared to the MCF technique[80]. However, larger tumors can cause stretch of the facial nerve and as such can increase its susceptibility to damage during surgery[80]. Furthermore, reports of post-operative headaches are more prevalent with the RS approach, in addition to a condition known as occipital pain syndrome[80].

*Translabyrinthine*

The final, and ultimately the most destructive technique, is the translabyrinthine (TL) surgical approach. Given the level of involvement required as well as the intricate anatomy, it is not uncommon for the TL approach to be performed by a team of surgeons[17]. The procedure is typically used for patients with larger tumors, patients who have poor hearing, or patients who have hearing that is not likely to be saved during surgery[80]. Because of the access provided by the TL approach, any size of tumor can be removed[68]. While this technique does allow for the most direct route to the area where the tumor is likely to occur, the surgical route taken also destroys the inner ear on the affected side. Consequently, hearing and balance perception is completely eliminated on the side that holds the tumor when using the TL approach[80]. This in turn requires that the patient's opposite inner ear will need to be relied upon for these functions.

Whereas hearing is eliminated on the affected side with the TL approach, preservation of facial nerve function becomes a main focal point. Like the RS approach, a successful TL surgery is often dependent upon size of the acoustic neuroma. Smaller neuromas (<2.5cm) resulted in 80% of patients retaining normal or slightly affected facial nerve function, while patients with tumors larger than 2.5cm maintained facial nerve function just 53% of the time[115].

*Sub-total tumor removal*

Patients undergoing surgery should not expect that the surgery will result in precise removal of the entire tumor. In fact, in some acoustic neuroma cases, complete removal of the tumor may not even be warranted. Such cases may occur with the elderly, in a patient who has some hearing still remaining in his or her 'good' ear, or in a patient where even partial tumor removal helps relieve compression on the brainstem and/or facial nerve function[17]. Other, potentially unexpected reasons for less than total removal of a tumor can include extensive surgical bleeding during a procedure, adherence of the tumor to structures such as the brain stem or facial nerve, or even swelling of structures in the brain during the surgery[72]. Still, even partial removal of the acoustic neuroma can help prevent further associated symptoms[116, 117].

While symptoms can typically be reduced after partial tumor removal, it does increase the possibility for tumor regrowth[118]. In fact, one study reported that if less than the entire tumor is removed during surgery, up to a nine-times greater chance for regrowth existed as compared to when the whole tumor is removed[119]. Even so, factors such as regrowth time, patient risk, and the degree of symptom reduction after removal should be factored in to a decision to remove less than the whole tumor.

Specific to regrowth, research indicates that when regrowth of an acoustic neuroma does occur after surgery, it typically does so within four years[120]. Unfortunately, follow-up for surgery for a tumor not fully removed originally has been shown to be a more difficult surgery, due in part to potentially altered positioning of structures in the skull which in turn require additional manipulation by the surgeon in order to complete the tumor removal[72]. But partial removal of a tumor is not the only reason for regrowth, as even total tumor removal can experience regrowth in 1-2% of cases[17].

## Conclusion

We have made tremendous advancements in not only the treatment of acoustic neuroma, but also in the success of those treatments. And as we continue to improve aspects such as surgical and treatment techniques, the involved technology, and the experience of those who diagnose these neuromas, there is no reason not to expect further improvements. At present, a shift toward conservative management is common for many neuromas, while larger or more debilitating neuromas are more likely to receive radiative therapy or surgery. Factors involved in the selection of the most appropriate treatment for a neuroma are many, and can include a patient's hearing status, the neuroma size and location, and the degree of symptoms that a patient is experiencing. In some cases, the patient may simply prefer a more aggressive treatment as opposed to 'waiting out' a tumor that is passively growing within his or her ear. Now, given the improvements in treatment options for patients, we'll next take a look at how an individual's quality of life is both affected by acoustic neuroma, along with outlining how one's life can improve with successful treatment.

# Chapter 5 – Quality of Life

When it comes to being a patient, having a particular disease is only one part of the equation. How that disease affects you as a patient as well as those around you is a whole other aspect that must be accounted for and may even play a role in when and what type of treatment you select. The degree to which an individual is affected by his or her particular disease is outlined by what is known as *quality of life*. If, for example, a disease does not impact a patient's own standards for health, comfort, or happiness in their life, that disease is said to have no real impact on quality of life. On the other hand, if a disease limits a patient's social interaction, or causes pain throughout the day, or prevents them from doing things like making their own breakfast, that disease likely has a significant impact on the respective patient's quality of life.

No matter the degree of injury or illness, the effect that a disease can have on an individual's quality of life is largely dependent upon a patient's own perception of that disease. For example, a retiree afflicted with vestibular attacks may report a much higher quality of life than a single mom trying to support her child by working two jobs in between a similar degree of vestibular attacks. Even if their degree of disability is the same, the impact that the attacks can have is likely higher for the single mom, thereby causing her to have a lower perceived quality of life.

Few will argue that living with acoustic neuroma can have a profound impact on an individual's quality of life. In many cases, a patient's quality of life can influence the type of treatment selected for acoustic neuroma patients. To examine this, we'll take an in-depth look in this chapter at how acoustic neuroma has been shown to affect a patient's quality of life, with particular interest of how treatment can play a role in improving quality of life in these patients.

## Assessing quality of life

Given how personal perception can play a role in a patient's quality of life, it can be somewhat challenging to assess how an illness such as acoustic neuroma impacts daily life for a patient. Traditionally, quality of life is measured using patient surveys that have been tested and validated for accuracy. Unfortunately, given the variation between patients that can occur with acoustic neuroma (e.g. tumor size, symptoms, treatment type, etc.), it can be difficult to gather enough data to form an effective evaluation that can outline quality of life in response to specific treatments. Furthermore, if a very generic survey was used to collect information, as often occurs in vestibular-based research, the resulting data may not be specific enough to clarify how a particular disease impacts the patient. For example, the Short-Form 36 (SF-36) survey asks 36 questions related to overall quality of life measures, and is commonly used as an assessment across a variety of health conditions. While well-accepted within the research and medical community, the SF-36 is not specific to acoustic neuroma. However, certain parts of the survey could be considered relevant to what acoustic neuroma patients deal with on a daily basis. such as the impact of the condition on the patient's ability to work or enjoy social functions[121].

Surveys are often refined or combined with other surveys to help draw out the most pertinent aspects of a particular medical condition. When this occurs, it is important to have the modified survey *validated* to ensure that it is both understandable to the patient and capable of capturing valid information. In recent years, a survey has been developed and validated specifically for acoustic neuroma patients. Called the Penn Acoustic Neuroma Quality-of-Life Scale (PANQOL), the survey evaluates several aspects of the disease including hearing, balance, facial nerve function, pain, anxiety, and health on a scale of 0-100[122]. Now, acoustic neuroma patients have the advantage of a targeted, disease-specific survey to help better outline how their lives are affected by this condition. Hopefully, this survey can be used to produce some viable and beneficial data specific to the impact of acoustic neuroma as well as how various treatments can affect a patient's quality of life.

## Patient vs. Physician Outcomes

As we discussed in the previous chapter, one of the main goals in the modern-day treatment of acoustic neuroma is not necessarily to remove the neuroma as much as to improve the patient's quality of life, particularly with minimal complications[123]. This is especially relevant given the shift toward more conservative treatment options rather than any attempt at removal or irradiation of the tumor. And given the shift towards conservative treatment, patients found to have even small tumors have been able to avoid unnecessary or complication-ridden surgery, instead dealing only with aspects such as diminished hearing or perhaps some degree of tinnitus. From a quality of life viewpoint, it would not be unexpected to find that most patients would rather accept a slight bit of hearing loss or tinnitus over time that comes with conservative (i.e. 'watch and wait') treatment as compared to the extensive rehabilitation of a RS surgery, or a significant loss of facial function due to damage of the facial nerve during a surgery that could potentially have waited ten or more years. The resulting psychological, physical, and even financial consequences of treatment are all important aspects to consider when assessing quality of life specific to acoustic neuroma.

Until just the past 20 years or so, many treatment strategies have focused on what is known as physician-centered outcomes – those factors that medical professionals are typically interested in such as hearing preservation, change in tumor size, nerve function, etc.[124]. In recent decades, however, treatment decisions have had much more patient input specific to what the patient feels is important such as recovery time, driving ability, or future quality of life issues. In separating physician-centered outcomes from those that are patient-centered, it helps point out that what a physician might see as effective treatment may not always match the patient's expectations simply because the anticipated outcomes are different[124]. For example, a physician may elect to observe a tumor's growth over time while a patient may not want the stress of knowing a tumor is growing within their skull and therefore opt for radiative treatment. Or a physician may feel that a tumor is in a prime location for surgical removal but the patient can't afford to take the required recovery time off from work.

While conflicts between a patient and his or her physician can occur, it should not be expected to be the norm. Rather, patients are often willing to go with the recommended treatment at the cost of some degree of impact on their quality of life as opposed to doing nothing and having more severe consequences down the road[81]. Even so, surgeons and physicians may still come across the occasional patient that is not happy with their treatment despite what the professional sees as an exceptional medical outcome[124].

## Quality of life with acoustic neuroma

Having an acoustic neuroma can be associated with several negative events. For example, hearing has been shown to deteriorate over time in response to the presence of acoustic neuroma. Despite this, the slow loss of hearing does not seem to have much impact on the patient's quality of life except for when a patient with complete hearing loss is in a social situation[125]. This finding is important, as attempts to remove or aggressively treat a tumor just to preserve a patient's remaining hearing will likely have much more negative impact – even if only in the short-term – on a patient's quality of life than what they could expect to have from the normal loss of hearing over time.

While hearing loss over time has been shown to have little impact on quality of life when it comes to acoustic neuroma, a much more prevalent impact occurs in patients who report vertigo. As we will discuss in the next chapter, acoustic neuroma is similar to many other vestibular conditions (e.g. Ménière's, vestibular migraine) in that vertigo is a common symptom. And for many of these other conditions, vertigo is often reported to have the most significant impact on quality of life, much like what has been shown to occur in acoustic neuroma patients[32]. In fact, the same acoustic neuroma patients that report a significant impact of vertigo on quality of life did not indicate any reduced quality of life due to hearing loss or tinnitus, which emphasizes the influence that vertigo can have on an individual's quality of life[32].

*Treatment options*

One of the remarkable aspects of any field of study is that it is always improving. But in order for anything to improve, we also have to know what *doesn't* work, or what can make a particular situation worse. In the case of medicine's view of acoustic neuroma, we used to think that surgical treatment was the best option, largely because by the time a neuroma was found it was already quite large and most likely causing significant disruption to the patient's life. Now, with our ability to use imaging to both detect smaller neuromas and monitor their growth over time, surgical intervention is not the priority it was many years ago.

Along the same lines, when reviewing acoustic neuroma studies on quality of life that are maybe 20 or even 30 years old, the techniques of that time must be taken into account. Because medicine is constantly improving, it's possible that any technique still used today has been improved upon since it was first studied, and as a result may produce more favorable outcomes now than even just a decade ago. As such, it is important to make the effort to use the most recent research available when assessing how a particular treatment may impact quality of life.

Take for example, surgical removal of an acoustic neuroma and its impact on quality of life. One study from 20 years ago looked at this relationship[126] and concluded that, as might be expected, acoustic neuroma surgery has a significant impact on one's quality of life. But there was no consistency among patients as to whether the surgery improved or worsened their quality of life. 54% of patients reported a worse overall quality of life post-surgery while the remainder indicated that they were the same or better. And the researchers found that tumor size did not have an impact on post-operative quality of life. This is important, because these findings clarify that the size of an individual's tumor prior to surgery should not be expected to influence their quality of life post-surgery.

With the emergence of conservative treatment as well as radiosurgery, acoustic neuroma patients now have additional options other than surgery. Conservative treatment should not be expected to have much impending change in a patient's quality of life as no procedure actually occurs on the patient. Radiosurgery appears to have very good effects on quality of life. In fact, radiosurgery patients are typically able to resume daily activity within 12 hours of the procedure[96]. There may be some lingering symptoms including imbalance or disequilibrium, but these are generally mild in nature and are usually minimized with small lifestyle adjustments[96].

As mentioned earlier, the PANQOL survey was developed specifically for acoustic neuroma patients[122]. Researchers found that patients who underwent surgery scored highest on the survey in what they called 'general' quality of life but scored lower in aspects such as hearing, facial nerve function, pain, and energy than both conservative and radiosurgery patients[127]. However, patients who underwent either stereotactic radiosurgery or surgery reported more similar – but lower overall – quality of life scores than those who underwent conservative treatment.

When looking at surgery for the treatment of acoustic neuroma, one of the major factors that can influence quality of life after the procedure is the loss of function of the facial nerve[81]. As we discussed in Chapter 2, the facial nerve is largely responsible for our ability to project facial expressions and also plays minor roles in aspects such as taste perception. Therefore, any facial nerve function that is lost due to the presence of an acoustic neuroma – or due to surgical intervention that in turn affects the facial nerve – can be expected to have a negative influence on a patient's quality of life.

While the research does indicate that surgery for acoustic neuroma can negatively affect quality of life, one study reviewed several research articles in order to compare the quality of life impact between radiosurgery and surgery. The researchers found that surgery decreased patient quality of life as much as 45% whereas radiosurgery showed a maximal decrease of 26%[55]. This is of importance for acoustic neuroma patients given that radiosurgery has been shown to have a more favorable preservation of hearing, have fewer complications from the surgery, and requires a shorter hospital stay[98]. And not only has radiosurgery been reported to provide a better quality of life than surgery, a separate study even reported that radiosurgery offered improved quality of life over conservative treatment as well[128]! Still, the decision as to which treatment is best must be a decision made between the patient and his or her physician, as there are multiple elements to take into account when making treatment decisions.

*Non-physical quality of life aspects*

Perhaps too often, quality of life emphasizes the potential for physical impairment or function. Doing so, however, tends to ignore other important factors that can affect an individual. Aspects such as psychological factors, financial impact, and social interference can also be affected by acoustic neuroma as well as its treatment. One study looked at some of these ancillary factors after surgery for acoustic neuroma, with interesting results[126]. Just under 30% of patients receiving surgery indicated that they became worse-off financially, and 21% had to change their occupation. Furthermore, tumor size had some degree of influence on financial status after the operation, with larger tumors being associated with a worse financial status. While probably not considered equivalent to physical complications by most patients, such results should be factored into a patient's treatment decision, particularly if he or she is the primary earner in the family or if they live in an area with limited job opportunities.

Aspects such as financial status must be viewed within the context of the patient when considering treatment options. For example, older acoustic neuroma patients have reported a better post-operation financial situation[126]. This improved situation could be impacted by issues such as retirement status or perhaps because older individuals were better established in their occupation and therefore may have had less complications resulting from any job-related impact of their acoustic neuroma. Therefore, when assessing quality of life data, the acoustic neuroma patient must be able to factor in these specifics (e.g. age, financial status, etc.) when making their treatment decisions.

# Therapy to improve quality of life

When it comes to improving the symptoms of acoustic neuroma, there are treatment options other than the traditional conservative, radiosurgery, or surgery options. For example, vestibular rehabilitation has been shown to help improve quality of life[129]. Vestibular rehabilitation typically includes exercises and activities that have been shown to improve symptoms related to many of the prevalent vestibular disorders. Exercises can include those that work on posture, vision tracking, balance, or general fitness, and are dependent upon an individual's own situation that is established as part of a thorough evaluation by a vestibular-trained professional.

As we discussed in the previous chapter, there are many treatment options for acoustic neuroma patients. Certainly, a diagnosis of acoustic neuroma can be expected to result in significant anxiety for a patient, which in turn can lead to a temporary reduction in their overall quality of life[130]. But it is of interest to note that an initial six-month observation period, during which tumor activity is monitored, has shown to generate a better anxiety-related quality of life score than among individuals who are newly diagnosed. While this difference is likely due to the fact that over those six months the patients have had time to cope with the news of their acoustic neuroma, it is important to highlight that perceived quality of life can be affected by time even when no treatment is applied to acoustic neuroma patients.

## Conclusion

Life with acoustic neuroma has improved tremendously from that experienced a century ago. Now, acoustic neuroma is not only recognized earlier but the neuroma is often left untouched until its presence causes significant harm or interference with the patient's daily life. When steps are taken to intervene, the outcomes now indicate a much more favorable quality of life post-intervention, even when the more invasive surgical approach is used. As research continues to progress and new technologies and techniques are developed, quality of life can be expected to continue to improve – hopefully to the point that acoustic neuroma becomes nothing more than an afterthought or a brief inconvenience in an otherwise productive life. Now, we'll take a look at several other medical conditions that often mimic the symptoms of acoustic neuroma. In doing so, we'll highlight not only the similarities between acoustic neuroma and these conditions but also provide evidence as to some of the differences that exist between these conditions as well.

# Chapter 6 – Related Conditions

Vestibular-related symptoms come in many shapes and sizes and are all capable of causing significant disability for the patient. The symptoms associated with acoustic neuroma often resemble those found with other inner-ear conditions, and as such it is of interest to note the *differences* that can exist between the many vestibular conditions which can cause symptoms such as unsteadiness, tinnitus, or hearing loss. Therefore, this chapter is designed to outline some of the more common medical conditions that can mimic the signs and symptoms associated with acoustic neuroma. In doing so, it not only highlights the similarities with acoustic neuroma but also outlines some key differences that can help medical professionals isolate acoustic neuroma as a potential culprit behind a patient's symptoms.

# Ménière's disease

Ménière's disease is an illness thought to result from problems with the fluid regulation system of the inner ear. Ménière's patients typically experience an ongoing degree of unsteadiness and ear pressure or fullness intermixed with bouts of acute vertigo, nausea, and vomiting that can last several hours or more. Due in large part to the complexity and sensitivity of the vestibular system, Ménière's remains a complicated disease. While the acute vertigo attacks of Ménière's can be extremely debilitating, those attacks can be followed by months or years of almost no symptoms.

Several theorized causes of Ménière's have been proposed, including body water regulation issues, endolymph reabsorption anomalies, vascular abnormalities, and autoimmune factors. Of these possible causes, fluid regulation in the middle ear is considered to be one of the main triggers of Ménière's[131]. For example, water channels, which regulate the transport of water across membranes, have been implicated as a possible main cause of Ménière's[132]. This theory results from the idea that unexpected reductions or increases in the number of water channels can influence the balance of fluid on each side of a membrane, and any alteration in fluid balance can have negative consequences in the equilibrium system of the ear.

Similarly, some researchers suggest that Ménière's patients have a diminished capacity to regulate fluid within their inner ear[133]. Consequently, fluctuations in the inner ear fluid are not well tolerated in Ménière's patients. This is thought to lead to fluid imbalances that contribute to many of the symptoms encountered by Ménière's patients. Electrolytes such as sodium that are known to play a role in the body's fluid regulation are commonly restricted in Ménière's patients in order to reduce potential fluctuations within the middle ear.

Other theorized causes of Ménière's disease include autoimmune disorders[134], the herpes virus[135], cervical (i.e. neck) disorders[136] and stress[137]. Whereas no definitive cause of Ménière's has been discovered, it is vital that research continue to investigate these and all logical possibilities to determine the potential link and/or similarities between Ménière's and acoustic neuroma. At present there remains no cure for Ménière's, though symptoms can often be controlled through the aforementioned sodium restriction, medication, intratympanic steroid injection, and if necessary, surgical procedures on the middle ear.

# Benign positional paroxysmal vertigo

As we have discussed, one of the most common vertigo conditions seen in primary care is benign positional paroxysmal vertigo (BPPV)[138]. Despite the long name, each word plays a role in describing what occurs with the disease. Most patients with this relatively harmless (benign) condition describe sudden (i.e.

paroxysmal) bouts of vertigo that occur with certain positional-dependent head positions.

The mechanism involved in BPPV is thought to be due to the presence of loose crystals (i.e. otoliths) within the semicircular canals of the ear. As otoliths are not normally present within the semicircular canals, certain head movements cause the loose otoliths to contact the delicate hair cells of the semicircular canals, causing them to trigger and falsely indicate body motion when the head is in particular positions. For example, patients with BPPV often report short bouts of vertigo when looking upwards or rolling over in bed[139]. Furthermore, nausea and vomiting can occur with more severe cases such as *intractable BPPV*.

Diagnosis of BPPV typically involves a thorough medical history and evaluation along with manipulating the head in an attempt to reproduce the symptoms. Most commonly, the Dix-Hallpike maneuver is used to attempt to reproduce the symptoms of BPPV. For this procedure, the patient is seated on a table and their head position is manipulated while the patient is put through a series of specific body positions. Because the otoliths will typically induce nystagmus along with vertigo, the patient's eyes are observed for nystagmus along with any patient-reported vertigo. Results of the Dix-Hallpike test are relatively reliable, being able to correctly identify patients with BPPV 83% of the time while correctly excluding patients without BPPV 52% of the time[138].

For those patients testing positive for BPPV, vestibular rehabilitation as well as canalith repositioning (e.g. Epley maneuver) are relatively successful. Vestibular rehabilitation typically consists of a series of head and/or body motions which may involve fixation of the eye on a single point. Pharmaceutical treatments are not recommended for use in the treatment of BPPV as research has shown no benefit[140]. It is also possible that BBPV symptoms return.

# Vestibular migraine

Vestibular migraines are among the more common vestibular disorders, affecting up to 1% of the population[141, 142] and up to 11% of patients seeking treatment in dizziness-related clinics[143]. Vestibular migraines are also relatively common in children, having been reported to occur in nearly 3% of children aged 6-12 years of age[144]. Like Ménière's disease, vestibular migraine has no universally accepted definition, which can in turn limit recognition of vestibular migraines in affected patients. Only recently were the diagnostic criteria established which include the following[143].

1. Vestibular migraine

**A**. At least 5 episodes with vestibular symptoms of moderate or severe intensity, lasting 5 minutes to 72 hours

**B**. Current or previous history of migraine with or without aura according to the                    International Classification of Headache Disorders (ICHD)

**C**. One or more migraine features with at least 50% of the vestibular episodes:

– headache with at least two of the following characteristics: one sided location, pulsating quality, moderate or severe pain intensity, aggravation by routine physical activity

– photophobia and phonophobia

– visual aura

**D**. Not better accounted for by another vestibular or ICHD diagnosis

2. Probable vestibular migraine

**A**. At least 5 episodes with vestibular symptoms of moderate or severe intensity, lasting 5 min to 72 hours

**B**. Only one of the criteria B and C for vestibular migraine is fulfilled (migraine history or migraine features during the episode)

**C**. Not better accounted for by another vestibular or ICHD diagnosis

The predominant symptoms of vestibular migraine include vertigo in combination with headache, and these two symptoms often occur relatively close to each other[139]. Other symptoms can include transient hearing fluctuations[145], nausea, vomiting, and a sensitivity to motion sickness[143]. Some patients have reported triggering of their migraine in response to dehydration, lack of sleep, or certain foods, but the relationship between these characteristics and vestibular migraines has not been well-studied[143]. Evidence of effective treatment of vestibular migraines is limited. Patients who respond favorably to anti-migraine medication have occurred, but the evidence is lacking as to overall effectiveness[146].

# Vestibular neuritis

Vestibular neuritis is associated with vertigo, nausea, vomiting, and imbalance, and is thought to be due to viral inflammation of the vestibular nerve[147]. The condition is acute in nature with symptoms lasting from a few days to several weeks, but up to half of those suffering from vestibular neuritis can experience symptoms much longer[148]. Vestibular neuritis has been reported to account for nearly 10% of all dizziness-related medical visits[149]. Interestingly, viral epidemics trigger an increased incidence of vestibular neuritis, lending evidence to its likely inflammatory origins[150].

Patients exhibiting vestibular neuritis will present with acute, severe vertigo[139]. The most severe attacks can last for one to two days and then gradually subside over the following weeks. Motion may worsen the vertigo, and some patients experience nausea and vomiting in conjunction with the vertigo[139]. Additional symptoms often include nystagmus along with a walking pattern in which the patient tends to lean toward the affected ear's side.

Treatment of vestibular neuritis includes symptomatic care along with vestibular rehabilitation, which can begin as soon as tolerable after cessation of immediate symptoms[139]. Vestibular rehabilitation has been reported to be successful when compared against no therapy[151]. If vestibular neuritis is severe, short-term hospitalization may be required[139].

## Concussion

Even a hit to the head has the potential to cause significant vestibular-related symptoms, and many of these symptoms mimic what one would expect from acoustic neuroma. Concussion is a type of traumatic brain injury that most often results from a direct hit to the head or a type of injury (e.g. whiplash) that causes the brain to move rapidly within the skull. Concussions are not uncommon, with over 3 million concussions thought to occur per year in the United States[152]. The cause of concussion can vary by age, as children and older adults most commonly experience concussion as a result of falls, while in adults the most common cause is motor vehicle accidents[153]. Athletic participation, especially high-contact sports such as football, hockey, or boxing is also a common cause for concussion and even includes a separate classification as *sport-related concussion*.

Like many vestibular-related symptoms, imaging through x-ray, MRI, CT scan, etc. is relatively ineffective at diagnosing concussion. Therefore, diagnosis is typically reliant upon the patient's history, description of the event that caused the concussion, and their symptoms. The range of symptoms that can occur in response to concussion can vary but do have a close resemblance to many of the symptoms of acoustic neuroma. Typically, symptoms of concussion are classified into three areas – cognitive, emotional, and psychological. Cognitive symptoms include difficulty concentrating or thinking (i.e. 'brain fog') in addition to difficulty with information retention. Emotional symptoms of concussion can include irritability, sadness, or general nervousness. Physical symptoms probably have the most similarity to acoustic neuroma as they can include headache, blurry vision, nausea and/or vomiting, sensitivity to light or noise, and imbalance issues, among others[153]. With such similarity in symptoms between acoustic neuroma and concussion, particularly among athletes or those who are susceptible to head-trauma events, it is somewhat easy to understand how acoustic neuroma may initially be misinterpreted as a concussion event.

Treatment of concussion is generally successful at relieving the associated symptoms. One of the first lines of treatment for concussion is rest. This includes both cognitive rest such as avoiding or reducing tasks that require a significant amount of 'thinking' (e.g. homework, computer use, etc.) as well as physical rest that avoids strenuous activity. Avoidance of associated triggers such as bright lights and loud noise is also recommended[154].

One of the positive aspects of concussion is that, unlike many other vestibular conditions, proper treatment generally results in a full recovery. Some individuals do have extended symptoms (e.g. 3 or more months), but the majority of individuals who suffer a concussion have relief of symptoms in a week or less and are typically allowed to resume activity. Having a concussion can predispose an individual to having a future concussion, so care must be taken to limit the opportunity for future concussions to occur.

# Conclusion

Acoustic neuroma research and treatment has made immense strides since the condition was first recognized well over a century ago. Patients no longer have to sit back and accept a slow deterioration of balance and now can expect to live a very productive life, often with minimal interruption from the symptoms associated with acoustic neuroma. Given the knowledge we have attained over the years, it is now considered acceptable within the medical community to adopt a 'watch and wait' approach to treatment of the neuroma rather than engage in an immediate intervention as has been done traditionally.

Of all the vestibular-related books I have written, this one soon became one of the most confounding. Part of the reason for this may be that my other books were written about conditions that have much less medical history behind them compared to acoustic neuroma. As a recognized medical condition, acoustic neuroma has been written about and studied in medicine for well over

100 years.  Those 100-plus years of research have generated an immense amount of information that has been agreed with, disproven, validated, and/or improved upon over time.  Consequently, writing this book required wading through and interpreting an immense amount of research, much of which was at one time accepted but is now passed over in favor of more recent or relevant findings.  Still, some research from 50 years ago or more remains relevant even today, resulting in a wide fluctuation in the age of the available research that is still currently relied upon for outlining acoustic neuroma.

Another aspect that I found during my research for this book is that acoustic neuroma has a physical, recognizable mass of tissue that is largely responsible for most all of the related symptoms.  Other conditions such as vestibular migraine, vestibular neuritis, or Ménière's disease are largely theoretical when it comes to outlining the true cause of the associated symptoms.  As such, acoustic neuroma research is much more focused on the neuroma as the source of the symptoms whereas research associated with other vestibular conditions make a very broad sweep of all potential structures and events that could be causing the symptoms.  So even though the acoustic neuroma research is often much older, there is a lot more congruency in what we know about the true cause.  And because we know the main cause of the symptoms associated with acoustic neuroma, researchers can focus their efforts on better ways to treat or even cure the condition, which can in turn allow patients the opportunity to maintain a higher quality of life.

Unpredictability is a common thread amongst all vestibular conditions. For example, vestibular migraine and Ménière's patients may go months or years without an attack followed by several in succession. BPPV patients may remain symptom-free until they place their head in a very specific position. Despite the physical presence of a tumor, acoustic neuroma patients are also subjected to a degree of unpredictability in that that the tumor may grow, stay the same, shrink, grow then shrink, or a variety of other possibilities. This can be as encouraging as it can be frustrating because the fact remains that the patient just doesn't know what to expect in terms of what the neuroma will do. However, with the vast amount of research available we now know that observation may be the best option for many patients, with only periodic check-ins required in order to find out if the neuroma has continued to grow. For those that do experience tumor growth to the point that it becomes problematic, they are now afforded multiple treatment options which are continually being improved. And as our body of knowledge continues to improve, the patient will become the biggest beneficiary.

I hope that this book has been able to increase your understanding and knowledge of acoustic neuroma. The process of writing this book has been highly educational even for me, and my goal was always to take the available information and put it into a format that is both educational and understandable for you the patient.

Having suffered from multiple vestibular disorders myself, I know the frustration that can occur when symptoms arise, and I also know the helplessness that arises when you can't find the information that you seek, or when it is not presented in a clear way. As such, my intent was to lead you through the available research and develop this book as a guide to help you better understand the intricacies of acoustic neuroma.

In closing, I wish you well and the best of luck on your journey with acoustic neuroma. With the wealth of available options out there, I also hope that you are able to achieve the best quality of life possible.

# References

1.  Ekdale, E.G., *Form and function of the mammalian inner ear.* Journal of anatomy, 2016. **228**(2): p. 324-337.
2.  Schuknecht, H. and R. Ruby, *Cupulolithiasis*, in *Otophysiology.* 1973, Karger Publishers. p. 434-443.
3.  Barral, J.-P. and A. Croibier, *Manual therapy for the cranial nerves.* 2008: Churchill Livingstone.
4.  Kentala, E. and I. Pyykkö, *Clinical picture of vestibular schwannoma.* Auris Nasus Larynx, 2001. **28**(1): p. 15-22.
5.  Lawal, O. and D. Navaratnam, *Causes of Central Vertigo*, in *Diagnosis and Treatment of Vestibular Disorders.* 2019, Springer. p. 363-375.
6.  Peng, B., *Cervical vertigo: historical reviews and advances.* World neurosurgery, 2018. **109**: p. 347-350.
7.  Lee, A., *Diagnosing the cause of vertigo: a practical approach.* Hong Kong Med J, 2012. **18**(4): p. 327-32.
8.  Glover, J.C., *Vestibular System*, in *Encyclopedia of Neuroscience*, L.R. Squire, Editor. 2004, Academic Press: Oxford. p. 127-132.
9.  Stedman, T.L., *Stedman's medical dictionary for the health professions and nursing.* 2005: Lippincott Williams & Wilkins.
10. Khan, A.M., et al., *Impact of Vestibular Schwannomas on Cerebrospinal Fluid (CSF) Pathway.* Bangladesh Journal of Neurosurgery Vol, 2016. **6**(1).
11. Rosegay, H., *The Krause operations.* Journal of neurosurgery, 1992. **76**(6): p. 1032-1036.
12. Pellet, W., *History of vestibular schwannoma surgery*, in *Modern Management of Acoustic Neuroma.* 2008, Karger Publishers. p. 6-23.
13. Lin, E. and B. Crane, *The management and imaging of vestibular schwannomas.* American Journal of Neuroradiology, 2017. **38**(11): p. 2034-2043.
14. Gentry, L., et al., *Cerebellopontine angle-petromastoid mass lesions: comparative study of diagnosis with MR imaging and CT.* Radiology, 1987. **162**(2): p. 513-520.

15. Propp, J.M., et al., *Descriptive epidemiology of vestibular schwannomas.* Neuro-oncology, 2006. **8**(1): p. 1-11.

16. Jackler RK, *Acoustic Neuroma (Vestibular Schwannoma)*, in *Neurotology*, Jackler RK and Brackmann DE, Editors. 1994, Mosby. p. 729-786.

17. Kaye, A.H., R.J. Briggs, and A.P. Morokoff, *Acoustic neurinoma (vestibular schwannoma)*, in *Brain Tumors*. 2012, Elsevier. p. 518-569.

18. Tos, M. and J. Thomsen, *Proposal of classification of tumor size in acoustic neuroma surgery.* Acoustic Neuroma. Amsterdam, The Netherlands: Kugler Publications, 1992: p. 133-7.

19. Foley, R.W., et al., *Signs and symptoms of acoustic neuroma at initial presentation: an exploratory analysis.* Cureus, 2017. **9**(11).

20. Nikolopoulos, T.P., et al., *Acoustic neuroma growth: a systematic review of the evidence.* Otology & Neurotology, 2010. **31**(3): p. 478-485.

21. Schwartz, M.S. and L.M. Fisher, *Incidence and clinical characteristics of acoustic neuroma in Beverly Hills.* Skull Base, 2006. **16**(S 1): p. A040.

22. Kshettry, V.R., et al., *Incidence of vestibular schwannomas in the United States.* Journal of neuro-oncology, 2015. **124**(2): p. 223-228.

23. Hernanz-Schulman, M., et al., *Acoustic neuromas in children.* American journal of neuroradiology, 1986. **7**(3): p. 519-521.

24. Borck, W. and K. Zülch, *Über die Erkrankungshäufigkeit der Geschlechter an Hirngeschwülsten.* Zbl. Neurochir, 1951. **11**: p. 333-350.

25. Dastur, D.K., V. Lalitha, and V. Prabhakar, *Pathological analysis of intracranial space-occupying lesions in 1000 cases including children: part 1. Age, sex and pattern; and the tuberculomas.* Journal of the neurological sciences, 1968. **6**(3): p. 575-592.

26. Huang, W.-q., et al., *Statistical analysis of central nervous system tumors in China.* Journal of neurosurgery, 1982. **56**(4): p. 555-564.

27. Barker, D., R. Weller, and J. Garfield, *Epidemiology of primary tumours of the brain and spinal cord: a regional survey in southern England.* Journal of Neurology, Neurosurgery & Psychiatry, 1976. **39**(3): p. 290-296.

28. Kurland, L.T., et al., *The incidence of primary intracranial neoplasms in Rochester, Minnesota, 1935-1977.* Annals of the New York Academy of Sciences, 1982. **381**(1): p. 6-16.

29. Rowe, J., et al., *Gamma knife stereotactic radiosurgery for unilateral acoustic neuromas.* Journal of Neurology, Neurosurgery & Psychiatry, 2003. **74**(11): p. 1536-1542.

30. Schmalbrock, P., et al., *Assessment of internal auditory canal tumors: a comparison of contrast-enhanced T1-weighted and steady-state T2-weighted gradient-echo MR imaging.* American journal of neuroradiology, 1999. **20**(7): p. 1207-1213.

31. Baguley, D.M., et al., *The Clinical Characteristics of Tinnitus in Patients with Vestibular Schwannoma.* Skull Base, 2006. **16**(2): p. 49-58.

32. Breivik, C.N., et al., *Conservative management of vestibular schwannoma—a prospective cohort study: treatment, symptoms, and quality of life.* Neurosurgery, 2011. **70**(5): p. 1072-1080.

33. Yoshimoto, Y., *Systematic review of the natural history of vestibular schwannoma.* Journal of neurosurgery, 2005. **103**(1): p. 59-63.

34. Agrawal, Y., et al., *Predictors of vestibular schwannoma growth and clinical implications.* Otology & Neurotology, 2010. **31**(5): p. 807-812.

35. Smouha, E.E., et al., *Conservative management of acoustic neuroma: a meta-analysis and proposed treatment algorithm.* The Laryngoscope, 2005. **115**(3): p. 450-454.

36. Sterkers, O., et al., *Slow versus rapid growing acoustic neuromas.* Acoustic neuroma. Kugler, Amsterdam, 1992: p. 145-147.

37. Valvassori, G.E. and M. Guzman, *Growth rate of acoustic neuromas.* The American journal of otology, 1989. **10**(3): p. 174-176.

38. Stangerup, S.-E., et al., *The natural history of vestibular schwannoma.* Otology & neurotology, 2006. **27**(4): p. 547-552.

39. Kondziolka, D., et al., *The newly diagnosed vestibular schwannoma: radiosurgery, resection, or observation?* Neurosurgical focus, 2012. **33**(3): p. E8.

40. Tschudi, D.C., T.E. Linder, and U. Fisch, *Conservative management of unilateral acoustic neuromas.* Otology & Neurotology, 2000. **21**(5): p. 722-728.

41. Nedzelski, J., et al., *Is no treatment good treatment in the management of acoustic neuromas in the elderly?* The Laryngoscope, 1986. **96**(8): p. 825-829.

42. Charabi, S., et al., *Acoustic neuroma (vestibular schwannoma): growth and surgical and nonsurgical consequences of the wait-and-see policy.* Otolaryngology—Head and Neck Surgery, 1995. **113**(1): p. 5-14.

43. Tan, T., *Non-contrast high resolution fast spin echo magnetic resonance imaging of acoustic schwannoma.* Singapore medical journal, 1999. **40**(1): p. 27-31.

44. Stangerup, S.-E., et al., *Long-term hearing preservation in vestibular schwannoma.* Otology & Neurotology, 2010. **31**(2): p. 271-275.

45. Roche, P.-H., et al., *The wait and see strategy for intracanalicular vestibular schwannomas,* in *Modern Management of Acoustic Neuroma.* 2008, Karger Publishers. p. 83-88.

46. Sughrue, M.E., et al., *The natural history of untreated sporadic vestibular schwannomas: a comprehensive review of hearing outcomes.* Journal of neurosurgery, 2010. **112**(1): p. 163-167.

47. Nedzelski, J., et al., *Conservative management of acoustic neuromas.* Otolaryngologic Clinics of North America, 1992. **25**(3): p. 691-705.

48. Nagano, O., et al., *Transient expansion of vestibular schwannoma following stereotactic radiosurgery.* Journal of neurosurgery, 2008. **109**(5): p. 811-816.

49. Preston-Martin, S., et al., *Noise trauma in the aetiology of acoustic neuromas in men in Los Angeles County, 1978-1985.* British journal of cancer, 1989. **59**(5): p. 783.

50. Berkowitz, O., et al., *Epidemiology and environmental risk factors associated with vestibular schwannoma.* World neurosurgery, 2015. **84**(6): p. 1674-1680.

51. Children's Tumor Foundation. *Neurofibromatosis.* Available from: https://www.ctf.org/images/uploads/documents/Neurofibromatosis-FAQs-Brochure.pdf.

52. Fong, B., et al., *The molecular biology and novel treatments of vestibular schwannomas: a review.* Journal of neurosurgery, 2011. **115**(5): p. 906-914.

53. Bebin, J., *Pathophysiology of acoustic tumors. Diagnosis.* 1979, Baltimore: University Park Press.

54. Stangerup, S.-E., et al., *Increasing annual incidence of vestibular schwannoma and age at diagnosis.* The Journal of Laryngology & Otology, 2004. **118**(8): p. 622-627.

55. Wolbers, J.G., et al., *What intervention is best practice for vestibular schwannomas? A systematic review of controlled studies.* BMJ open, 2013. **3**(2): p. e001345.

56. Johnson, E., *Auditory test results in 500 cases of acoustic neuroma.* Archives of Otolaryngology, 1977. **103**(3): p. 152-158.

57. Hardy, D.G., et al., *Facial nerve recovery following acoustic neuroma surgery.* British journal of neurosurgery, 1989. **3**(6): p. 675-680.

58. Arribas, L., et al., *Non surgical treatment of vestibular schwannoma.* Acta Otorrinolaringologica (English Edition), 2015. **66**(4): p. 185-191.

59. Arthurs, B.J., et al., *A review of treatment modalities for vestibular schwannoma.* Neurosurgical review, 2011. **34**(3): p. 265-279.

60. Lee, S.H., et al., *Otologic manifestations of acoustic neuroma.* Acta oto-laryngologica, 2015. **135**(2): p. 140-146.

61. Hajioff, D., et al., *Conservative management of vestibular schwannomas: third review of a 10-year prospective study.* Clinical Otolaryngology, 2008. **33**(3): p. 255-259.

62. Sataloff, R.T., B. Davies, and D.L. Myers, *Acoustic neuromas presenting as sudden deafness.* The American journal of otology, 1985. **6**(4): p. 349-352.

63. Shaia, F.T. and J.L. Sheehy, *Sudden sensori-neural hearing impairment: A report of 1,220 cases.* The Laryngoscope, 1976. **86**(3): p. 389-398.

64. Day, A.-S., et al., *Correlating the cochleovestibular deficits with tumor size of acoustic neuroma.* Acta otolaryngologica, 2008. **128**(7): p. 756-760.

65. Nadol, J.J., P.F. Diamond, and A.R. Thornton, *Correlation of hearing loss and radiologic dimensions of vestibular schwannomas (acoustic Neuromas).* The American journal of otology, 1996. **17**(2): p. 312-316.

66. Roosli, C., et al., *Dysfunction of the cochlea contributing to hearing loss in acoustic neuromas: an underappreciated entity.* Otology & neurotology: official publication of the American Otological Society, American Neurotology Society [and] European Academy of Otology and Neurotology, 2012. **33**(3): p. 473.

67. von Kirschbaum, C. and R. Gürkov, *Audiovestibular function deficits in vestibular schwannoma.* BioMed Research International, 2016. **2016**.

68. Mowat, A., *The Management of Vestibular Schwannoma in the 21st Century.* Vol. 04. 2017.

69. Samii, M. and C. Matthies, *Management of 1000 vestibular schwannomas (acoustic neuromas): the facial nerve-preservation and restitution of function.* Neurosurgery, 1997. **40**(4): p. 684-695.

70. Kohno, M., et al., *Prognosis of tinnitus after acoustic neuroma surgery—surgical management of postoperative tinnitus.* World neurosurgery, 2014. **81**(2): p. 357-367.

71. Koos, W., *Microsurgery of cerebellopontine angle tumors.* Clinical microneurosurgery, 1976.

72. Jung, G. and R. Ramina, *Vestibular Schwannomas: Diagnosis and Surgical Treatment*, in *Primary Intracranial Tumors.* 2019, IntechOpen.

73. Choi, K.-S., et al., *Preoperative identification of facial nerve in vestibular schwannomas surgery using diffusion tensor tractography.* Journal of Korean Neurosurgical Society, 2014. **56**(1): p. 11.

74. Dix, M., *The vestibular acoustic system.* Handbook of Clinical Neurology, 1974. **16**: p. 301-340.

75. Boesen, T., et al. *Papilledema in patients with acoustic neuromas: vestibular and other oto-neurosurgical findings.* in *First International Conference on Acoustic Neuroma.* 1991. Copenhagen Denmark.

76. Borgmann, H., T. Lenarz, and M. Lenarz, *Preoperative prediction of vestibular schwannoma's nerve of origin with posturography and electronystagmography.* Acta oto-laryngologica, 2011. **131**(5): p. 498-503.

77. Tringali, S., et al., *Characteristics of 629 vestibular schwannomas according to preoperative caloric responses.* Otology & Neurotology, 2010. **31**(3): p. 467-472.

78. Ushio, M., et al., *Is the nerve origin of the vestibular schwannoma correlated with vestibular evoked myogenic potential, caloric test, and auditory brainstem response?* Acta oto-laryngologica, 2009. **129**(10): p. 1095-1100.

79. Musiek, F.E., et al., *ABR results in patients with posterior fossa tumors and normal pure-tone hearing.* Otolaryngology—Head and Neck Surgery, 1986. **94**(6): p. 568-573.

80. Basura, G.J., C. Budenz, and H.A. Arts, *Vestibular Schwannomas: Surgical and Nonsurgical Management.* Current Surgery Reports, 2015. **3**(3): p. 5.

81. Harati, A., et al., *Clinical features, microsurgical treatment, and outcome of vestibular schwannoma with brainstem compression.* Surgical neurology international, 2017. **8**.

82. Bess, F.H., et al., *Audiologic manifestations in bilateral acoustic tumors (von Recklinghausen's disease).* Journal of Speech and Hearing Disorders, 1984. **49**(2): p. 177-182.

83. Myrseth, E., et al., *Vestibular schwannoma: surgery or gamma knife radiosurgery? A prospective, nonrandomized study.* Neurosurgery, 2009. **64**(4): p. 654-663.

84. Patel, J., et al., *The changing face of acoustic neuroma management in the USA: analysis of the 1998 and 2008 patient surveys from the acoustic neuroma association.* British journal of neurosurgery, 2014. **28**(1): p. 20-24.

85. Martin, T.P., et al., *Conservative versus primary surgical treatment of acoustic neuromas: a comparison of*

*rates of facial nerve and hearing preservation.* Clinical Otolaryngology, 2008. **33**(3): p. 228-235.

86. Suryanarayanan, R., et al., *Vestibular schwannoma: role of conservative management.* The Journal of Laryngology & Otology, 2010. **124**(3): p. 251-257.

87. Pennings, R.J.E., et al., *Natural history of hearing deterioration in intracanalicular vestibular schwannoma.* Neurosurgery, 2011. **68**(1): p. 68-77.

88. Walsh, R., et al., *The role of conservative management of vestibular schwannomas.* Clinical Otolaryngology & Allied Sciences, 2000. **25**(1): p. 28-39.

89. Hoistad, D.L., et al., *Update on conservative management of acoustic neuroma.* Otology & neurotology, 2001. **22**(5): p. 682-685.

90. MacKeith, S.A., R.S. Kerr, and C.A. Milford, *Trends in acoustic neuroma management: a 20-year review of the oxford skull base clinic.* Journal of Neurological Surgery Part B: Skull Base, 2013. **74**(04): p. 194-200.

91. Woodson, E.A., et al., *Long-term hearing preservation after microsurgical excision of vestibular schwannoma.* Otology & neurotology: official publication of the American Otological Society, American Neurotology Society [and] European Academy of Otology and Neurotology, 2010. **31**(7): p. 1144.

92. Niranjan, A., et al., *Hearing preservation after intracanalicular vestibular schwannoma radiosurgery.* Neurosurgery, 2008. **63**(6): p. 1054-1063.

93. Régis, J., et al., *Functional outcome after gamma knife surgery or microsurgery for vestibular schwannomas.* Journal of neurosurgery, 2002. **97**(5): p. 1091-1100.

94. Misra, B.K., et al., *Current treatment strategy in the management of vestibular schwannoma.* Neurology India, 2009. **57**(3): p. 257.

95. Niranjan, A., E. Monaco, and L.D. Lunsford, *27 - Complications in Vestibular Schwannoma Patients*, in *Complications in Neurosurgery*, A. Nanda, Editor. 2019, Content Repository Only!: London. p. 141-147.

96. Niranjan, A., D. Kondziolka, and L.D. Lunsford, *Neoplastic transformation after radiosurgery or radiotherapy: risk and realities.* Otolaryngologic clinics of North America, 2009. **42**(4): p. 717-729.

97. Seferis, C., et al., *Malignant transformation in vestibular schwannoma: report of a single case, literature search, and debate: Case report.* Journal of neurosurgery, 2014. **121**(Suppl_2): p. 160-166.

98. Pollock, B.E., et al., *Patient outcomes after vestibular schwannoma management: a prospective comparison of microsurgical resection and stereotactic radiosurgery.* Neurosurgery, 2006. **59**(1): p. 77-85.

99. Milligan, B.D., et al., *Long-term tumor control and cranial nerve outcomes following gamma knife surgery for larger-volume vestibular schwannomas.* Journal of neurosurgery, 2012. **116**(3): p. 598-604.

100. Patel, T.R. and V.L. Chiang, *Secondary neoplasms after stereotactic radiosurgery.* World neurosurgery, 2014. **81**(3-4): p. 594-599.

101. Pollock, B.E., et al., *The risk of radiation-induced tumors or malignant transformation after single-fraction intracranial radiosurgery: results based on a 25-year experience.* International Journal of Radiation Oncology* Biology* Physics, 2017. **97**(5): p. 919-923.

102. Tamura, M., et al., *Hearing preservation after gamma knife radiosurgery for vestibular schwannomas presenting with high-level hearing.* Neurosurgery, 2009. **64**(2): p. 289-296.

103. Lunsford, L.D., et al., *Radiosurgery of vestibular schwannomas: summary of experience in 829 cases.* Journal of neurosurgery, 2005. **102**(Special_Supplement): p. 195-199.

104. Link, M.J., et al., *Radiation Therapy and Radiosurgery for Vestibular Schwannomas:: Indications, Techniques, and Results.* Otolaryngologic Clinics of North America, 2012. **45**(2): p. 353-366.

105. Brackmann, D.E., et al., *Prognostic factors for hearing preservation in vestibular schwannoma surgery.* Otology & Neurotology, 2000. **21**(3): p. 417-424.

106. Hillman, T., et al., *Facial nerve function and hearing preservation acoustic tumor surgery: does the approach matter?* Otolaryngology--Head and Neck Surgery, 2010. **142**(1): p. 115-119.

107. Staecker, H., et al., *Hearing preservation in acoustic neuroma surgery: middle fossa versus retrosigmoid*

*approach.* Otology & Neurotology, 2000. **21**(3): p. 399-404.

108. Noudel, R., et al., *Hearing preservation and facial nerve function after microsurgery for intracanalicular vestibular schwannomas: comparison of middle fossa and restrosigmoid approaches.* Acta neurochirurgica, 2009. **151**(8): p. 935.

109. Arriaga, M.A., W.M. Luxford, and K.I. Berliner, *Facial nerve function following middle fossa and translabyrinthine acoustic tumor surgery: a comparison.* The American journal of otology, 1994. **15**(5): p. 620-624.

110. Fayad, J.N. and D.E. Brackmann, *Treatment of small acoustic tumors (vestibular schwannomas).* Neurosurgery Quarterly, 2005. **15**(2): p. 127-137.

111. Phillips, D.J., et al., *Predictive factors of hearing preservation after surgical resection of small vestibular schwannomas.* Otology & Neurotology, 2010. **31**(9): p. 1463-1468.

112. Elhammady, M.S., F.F. Telischi, and J.J. Morcos, *Retrosigmoid approach: indications, techniques, and results.* Otolaryngologic Clinics of North America, 2012. **45**(2): p. 375-97, ix.

113. Sughrue, M.E., et al., *Preservation of facial nerve function after resection of vestibular schwannoma.* British journal of neurosurgery, 2010. **24**(6): p. 666-671.

114. Zhao, X., et al., *Long-term facial nerve function evaluation following surgery for large acoustic neuromas via retrosigmoid transmeatal approach.* Acta neurochirurgica, 2010. **152**(10): p. 1647-1652.

115. Brackmann, D.E., R.D. Cullen, and L.M. Fisher, *Facial nerve function after translabyrinthine vestibular schwannoma surgery.* Otolaryngology—Head and Neck Surgery, 2007. **136**(5): p. 773-777.

116. Olivecrona, H., *Acoustic tumors.* Journal of neurosurgery, 1967. **26**(1part1): p. 6-13.

117. Wazen, J., et al., *Preoperative and postoperative growth rates in acoustic neuromas documented with CT scanning.* Otolaryngology—Head and Neck Surgery, 1985. **93**(2): p. 151-155.

118. Hitselberger, W. and W. House, *Partial versus total removal of acoustic tumors.* Acoustic Tumors, 1979. **2**: p. 265-268.

119. Carlson, M.L., et al., *Magnetic resonance imaging surveillance following vestibular schwannoma resection.* The Laryngoscope, 2012. **122**(2): p. 378-388.

120. House, W.F., *Partial tumor removal and recurrence in acoustic tumor surgery.* Archives of Otolaryngology, 1968. **88**(6): p. 644-654.

121. Instrument Ware Jr, J. and C. Sherbourne, *The MOS 36-item short-form health survey (SF-36): I. Conceptual framework and item selection.* Medical care, 1992. **30**(6): p. 473-483.

122. Shaffer, B.T., et al., *Validation of a disease-specific quality-of-life instrument for acoustic neuroma: The Penn Acoustic Neuroma Quality-of-Life Scale.* The Laryngoscope, 2010. **120**(8): p. 1646-1654.

123. Wu, H., et al., *Summary and consensus in 7th International Conference on acoustic neuroma: An update for the management of sporadic acoustic neuromas.* World journal of otorhinolaryngology-head and neck surgery, 2016. **2**(4): p. 234-239.

124. Carlson, M.L., et al., *Long-term quality of life in patients with vestibular schwannoma: an international multicenter cross-sectional study comparing microsurgery, stereotactic radiosurgery, observation, and nontumor controls.* Journal of neurosurgery, 2015. **122**(4): p. 833-842.

125. Gardner, G. and J.H. Robertson, *Hearing preservation in unilateral acoustic neuroma surgery.* Annals of Otology, Rhinology & Laryngology, 1988. **97**(1): p. 55-66.

126. Nikolopoulos, T.P., I. Johnson, and G.M. O'Donoghue, *Quality of life after acoustic neuroma surgery.* The Laryngoscope, 1998. **108**(9): p. 1382-1385.

127. McLaughlin, E.J., et al., *Quality of life in acoustic neuroma patients.* Otology & Neurotology, 2015. **36**(4): p. 653-656.

128. Whitmore, R.G., et al., *Decision analysis of treatment options for vestibular schwannoma.* Journal of neurosurgery, 2011. **114**(2): p. 400-413.
129. Lloyd, S.K., et al., *Audiovestibular factors influencing quality of life in patients with conservatively managed sporadic vestibular schwannoma.* Otology & Neurotology, 2010. **31**(6): p. 968-976.
130. Carlson, M.L., et al., *Quality of life within the first 6 months of vestibular schwannoma diagnosis with implications for patient counseling.* Otology & Neurotology, 2018. **39**(10): p. e1129-e1136.
131. Minor, L.B., D.A. Schessel, and J.P. Carey, *Meniere's disease.* Current opinion in neurology, 2004. **17**(1): p. 9-16.
132. Ishiyama, G., I. Lopez, and A. Ishiyama, *Aquaporins and Meniere's disease.* Current Opinion in Otolaryngology & Head and Neck Surgery, 2006. **14**(5): p. 332-336.
133. Rauch, S.D., *Clinical Hints and Precipitating Factors in Patients Suffering from Meniere's Disease.* Otolaryngologic Clinics of North America, 2010. **43**(5): p. 1011-1017.
134. Kangasniemi, E. and E. Hietikko, *The theory of autoimmunity in Meniere's disease is lacking evidence.* Auris Nasus Larynx, 2018. **45**(3): p. 399-406.
135. Vrabec, J.T., *Herpes simplex virus and Meniere's Disease.* The Laryngoscope, 2003. **113**(9): p. 1431-1438.
136. Bjorne, A., A. Berven, and G. Agerberg, *Cervical Signs and Symptoms in Patients with Meniere's Disease: A Controlled Study.* CRANIO®, 1998. **16**(3): p. 194-202.
137. Söderman, A.C.H., et al., *Stress as a Trigger of Attacks in Menière's Disease. A Case-Crossover Study.* The Laryngoscope, 2004. **114**(10): p. 1843-1848.
138. Hanley, K., *Symptoms of vertigo in general practice: a prospective study of diagnosis.* Br J Gen Pract, 2002. **52**(483): p. 809-812.
139. Wipperman, J., *Dizziness and vertigo.* Primary Care: Clinics in Office Practice, 2014. **41**(1): p. 115-131.

140. Bhattacharyya, N., et al., *Clinical practice guideline: benign paroxysmal positional vertigo.* Otolaryngology--Head and Neck Surgery, 2008. **139**(5_suppl): p. 47-81.
141. Cherchi, M. and T.C. Hain, *Migraine-associated vertigo.* Otolaryngologic Clinics of North America, 2011. **44**(2): p. 367-375.
142. Neuhauser, H., et al., *Migrainous vertigo Prevalence and impact on quality of life.* Neurology, 2006. **67**(6): p. 1028-1033.
143. Lempert, T., et al., *Vestibular migraine: diagnostic criteria.* Journal of Vestibular Research, 2012. **22**(4): p. 167-172.
144. Abu-Arafeh, I. and G. Russell, *Paroxysmal vertigo as a migraine equivalent in children: a population-based study.* Cephalalgia, 1995. **15**(1): p. 22-25.
145. Johnson, G.D., *Medical management of migraine-related dizziness and vertigo.* The Laryngoscope, 1998. **108**(S85): p. 1-28.
146. Fotuhi, M., et al., *Vestibular migraine: a critical review of treatment trials.* Journal of neurology, 2009. **256**(5): p. 711-716.
147. Schuknecht, H.F. and K. Kitamura, *Vestibular neuritis.* Annals of Otology, Rhinology & Laryngology, 1981. **90**(1_suppl): p. 1-19.
148. Perols, J.B., Olle, *Vestibular neuritis: a follow-up study.* Acta oto-laryngologica, 1999. **119**(8): p. 895-899.
149. Neuhauser, H.K. and T. Lempert. *Vertigo: epidemiologic aspects.* in *Seminars in neurology.* 2009. © Thieme Medical Publishers.
150. Baloh, R.W. and V. Honrubia, *Clinical neurophysiology of the vestibular system.* 2001: Oxford University Press, USA.
151. Hillier, S.L. and M. McDonnell, *Vestibular rehabilitation for unilateral peripheral vestibular dysfunction.* The Cochrane Library, 2011.
152. Brain Injury Research Institute. *What is a concussion?* ; Available from: http://www.protectthebrain.org/.
153. Centers for Disease Control and Prevention, *Traumatic Brain Injury and Concussion.* 2019.
154. Broglio, S.P., et al., *National Athletic Trainers' Association position statement: management of sport*

*concussion.* Journal of athletic training, 2014. **49**(2): p. 245-265.

# Resources for Acoustic Neuroma Patients

**Acoustic Neuroma Association**

http://www.anausa.org

**Vestibular Disorders Association**

https://vestibular.org/acoustic-neuroma

**MedlinePlus**

https://medlineplus.gov/acousticneuroma.html

**British Acoustic Neuroma Association**

https://www.bana-uk.com/

**Acoustic Neuroma Association of Canada**

https://www.anac.ca/

**American Brain Tumor Association**

https://www.abta.org/tumor_types/acousticneuroma/

# Let others know!

If you found this or any of Mark's other books informative, *please take the time and post a review online*! Reviews help get exposure for the books and thereby improve the chances that others will be able to benefit from the material as well!

## Check out these other books by Mark Knoblauch

*Challenge the Hand You Were Dealt: Strategies to battle back against adversity and improve your chances for success*

*Essentials of Writing and Publishing Your Self-Help Book*

*Living Low Sodium: A guide for understanding our relationship with sodium and how to be successful in adhering to a low-sodium diet*

*Outlining Tinnitus: A comprehensive guide to help you break free of the ringing in your ears*

*Overcoming Ménière's: How changing your lifestyle can change your life*

*Professional Writing in Kinesiology and Sports Medicine*

*Seven Ways To Make Running Not Suck*

*The Art of Efficiency: A guide for improving task management in the home to help maximize your leisure time*

*Understanding BPPV: Outlining the causes and effects of Benign Paroxysmal Positional Vertigo*

*Vestibular Migraine: A Comprehensive Patient Guide*

# About the Author

Mark is a small-town Kansas native who now lives in a suburb of Houston with his wife and two young daughters. His background is in the area of sports medicine, obtaining his bachelor's degree from Wichita State and his master's degree from the University of Nevada, Las Vegas. After working clinically as an athletic trainer for eight years, Mark returned to graduate school where he received his doctorate in Kinesiology from the University of Houston, followed by a postdoctoral assistantship in Molecular Physiology and Biophysics at Baylor College of Medicine in Houston, TX. He has been employed as a college professor at the University of Houston since 2013.

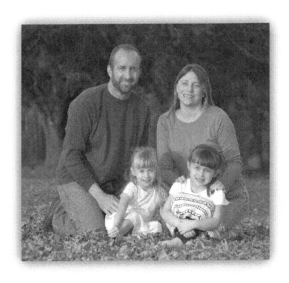

Made in the USA
Middletown, DE
28 March 2021